POLIO'S LEGACY

An Oral History

Edmund J. Sass
with
George Gottfried
Anthony Sorem

Foreword by
Richard Owen

University Press of America, Inc.
Lanham • New York • London

Copyright © 1996 by
University Press of America,® Inc.
4720 Boston Way
Lanham, Maryland 20706

3 Henrietta Street
London, WC2E 8LU England

Library of Congress Cataloging-in-Publication Data

Polio's legacy : an oral history / edited by Edmund J. Sass with George
Gottfried, Anthony Sorem ; foreword by Richard Owen.
p.   cm.
Includes bibliographical references.
1. Poliomyelitis--United States--Biography.   I. Sass, Edmund J. II.
Gottfried, George. III. Sorem, Anthony.
Rc181.U5P65   1996   616.8'35--dc20   95-45236 CIP

ISBN 0-7618-0143-X (cloth: alk: ppr.)
ISBN 0-7618-0144-8 (pbk: alk: ppr.)

Dedicated to the parents of polio survivors:

Though we went through hell, we took our parents along for the ride... and they never complained.

Contents

Foreword

Edmund Sass and his associates in the preparation of this oral history have done a great service in the bringing together and editing of poliomyelitis stories. This excellent book provides a history of an era from the 1930's to the early 1990's. The narratives it includes are individualized and personal and yet transcend that by representing, in most cases, shared experiences of acute illness, extended hospitalizations, and separation from family and friends. The book tells the story of an infectious disease of the central nervous system that was caused by a small organism called a virus and the physical, personal, and societal ramifications of that disease. In many ways, the stories are quite like those heard in a post-polio outpatient clinic. One great difference is the absence of leading or biased questioning on the part of the examining health professional. Some of the stories contain natural historical distortions based on the passage of time, imparted perceptions from family or friends, and miscommunication with health professionals. Offhanded descriptions of surgical or medical interventions by physicians often misled patients and their families about potential for successful outcome and/or complications. Misplaced optimism and desire for a return to "normal" often led to disappointment when the stitches were taken out, the cast removed, the new medicine tried, or the new brace applied.

Gradual and spontaneous improvement after the acute infection took place naturally over a two-year period during which a miraculous process of nerve-fiber sprouting occurred in an effort of the body to restore nerve supply to muscle fibers paralyzed by nerve cell damage. These changes of improved muscle functioning were often credited to or appeared to be related to treatment, exercise, and work. For many of us, the acute illness and convalescence was during adolescence with the impact of polio superimposed on all the usual stresses and strains of growing up. Barriers to buildings, activities, opportunities, and associations added to frustration and, in some cases, social isolation of young people with the residuals of poliomyelitis. Many barriers to a sense of integration were self-imposed. Various coping mechanisms often covered true feelings of loss. Denial often led to a distorted reality. Fantasy and other forms of escape provided temporary avoidance of painful experiences or expectations. Growth in height and weight and the resulting relocation of our bodies' centers of gravity increased disability in individuals with lower-extremity paralysis or scoliosis. Bracing and surgery often interfered with life activities and schedules. Family support and sacrifices in the provision of transportation, home exercises, and social development are common themes in many of the stories.

After the separation from family, friends, and usual life experiences, the person with polio residuals typically returned to the "mainstream" of life, school, society, and vocation. There was an extended period of relative stability. Except for periods of rehospitalization or outpatient clinic visits, people with polio were usually widely dispersed in society. There were no formal support groups although communication around the world was maintained by Gini Laurie whose *Rehabilitation Gazette* served as a clearinghouse for information about new experiences and techniques. She was particularly successful in keeping in touch with ventilator-dependent people.

Decay and loss of function were not expected. Some people with the late effects of polio experienced new disability, but the attention to these problems was scattered and not generally reported. Many of us in rehabilitation would see people requiring ventilator assistance in respiratory distress with intercurrent infections or loss of chest-wall flexibility. Overuse injury, fractures, or sprains often resulted in the need for extended periods of immobilization or physical therapy. Prescriptions for braces, wheelchairs, assistive devices, and handicapped parking permit applications required periodic brief visits to physicians. There had been no systematic review of activities of daily living, range of motion, or muscle tests. Changes in muscle function occurred slowly and subtly and went unnoticed by the post-polio person until a significant capability was lost such as climbing a curb, opening bottles, or getting in and out of chairs. In 1980, Drs. Lauro Halstead and David Wiechers became interested in this phenomenon and began to survey groups of people who had polio years earlier in an effort to discover if something new was happening and what was common within the group of people with post-polio problems.

In 1981, *Time Magazine* reported that 600,000 people who had had acute poliomyelitis years before were sitting on a "time bomb" with the potential to develop new problems very much like amyotrophic lateral sclerosis (ALS or Lou Gehrig's disease). This news item was about the emerging phenomenon of post-polio syndrome and the work of Gini Laurie of the *Rehabilitation Gazette* in planning a conference in Chicago. The subtitle of that meeting was the "Whatever Happened to the Old Polios Conference." Its purpose was to gather together scientists, physicians, health-care providers, people with polio residuals and their families, government officials, and the press on the subject of the new things happening to post-polio people for purposes of shared information, concern, support, and strategies to address these new difficulties. In 1974, Dr. Donald Mulder at the Mayo Clinic had written an article about the late progression of poliomyelitis. Others far earlier had described chronic poliomyelitis as a condition of late symptoms associated with an earlier attack of acute poliomyelitis. The conference was a powerful experience and a great success. A fascinating group of speakers and participants came together from around the world. There was a great variety of supporting technology displayed by the attendees ranging from iron lungs and curass ventilators to positive-pressure breathing machines; from heavy, metal-and-leather bracing to clean, lightweight plastic orthotics; and wheelchairs of every imaginable design and vintage.

The presenters spoke in alarming fashion of a process of progressive degeneration very similar to that experienced with ALS. In spite of this gloomy portent, the attendees were both excited and exciting in sharing experiences, insights, and coping mechanisms. Some spoke of a latent or lurking polio virus as the cause of post-polio syndrome. Dr. Maynard of the University of Michigan talked of "premature aging" in polio-affected muscles. He commented on looking out on a room of 50-year-olds with 90-year-old muscles. Other speakers emphasized the danger of overuse of weakened muscles as a probable cause of the new problems facing us.

When I returned to Minneapolis after the GINI conference, I started the Post-polio Clinic at the Sister Kenny Institute, and we had our first conference in Minneapolis in early 1982. Many of the patients we saw early in the Clinic at Sister Kenny Institute were experiencing a slow and gentle decline associated with aging, weight gain, change in lifestyle, other muscle or joint problems, intercurrent health issues, and a general reduction in physically challenging activities. We set up a protocol for evaluation and management based on traditional rehabilitation models and the concepts of polio management laid down by Elizabeth Kenny. Our first 20 patients evaluated for cardiac fitness were conditioned on the average at about a stage comparable to a person just two weeks out of a coronary care unit. This led to an adapted cardiopulmonary fitness program using intervals of exercise in order to facilitate adequate oxygen supply to involved muscles. As time passed, the origins and varieties of expressions of the syndrome suggested a number of different causative factors. Many people with polio residuals had neither been examined nor had a muscle test for 30 or 40 years. Some had old braces held together by haywire and solder. Most had not reconsidered or retold their histories and the interim experiences with disability, handicaps, and barriers for many years. Workshops and informational meetings became reunions of sorts and opportunities for the retelling of polio stories.

In 1984, The First Research Conference on the Late Effects of Poliomyelitis was held at Warm Springs, Georgia. This was sponsored by the Roosevelt Foundation headed by James Roosevelt. Experts in neuropathology, viral disease, aging, ventilation, rehabilitation, and research were brought together. Dr. David Bodian from Johns Hopkins University, the neuropathologist who defined the nature of the polio infection and had also shown the significant involvement of the lower portions of the brain in inflammation and degeneration, was very helpful in redefining for us the scope of the initial infection. His studies helped explain for many of us the nature of damage possible in post-polio subjects who had shown little or no significant paralysis at the time of acute infection. Dr. Richard Bruno and Nancy Frick believed that brain involvement contributed to some of the symptoms of pain, cold intolerance, and severe generalized fatigue in the post-polio syndrome. Many at the research conference recognized the significance of the research of Willis Beasley in "non-paralytic polios" at the Sister Kenny Institute in the 1950's. Dr. Beasley had found an average loss of almost 50% in calf muscle strength in a "non-paralytic" group as opposed to a "normal" population. That would represent a significant loss of motor cells in the spinal cord in individuals who were discharged as non-paralytic polios. This degree of motor loss explains the unexpected recurrence of weakness in some who had very little in the way of residuals from the acute attack of poliomyelitis but are now facing new polio-related problems. An interesting debate raged over the issue of exercise as opposed to rest. Dr. Reubin Feldman from the University of Alberta and I were the only proponents of a formalized exercise protocol. Both of us had come to the conclusion that injudicious exercise or sustained overwork (incidental exercise) of a repetitive maximum nature could damage polio-involved musculature, but a structured exercise program could be beneficial. Concern over a latent virus lurking in the spinal cord or an immunologic reaction in the central nervous system was voiced by a number of investigators. Debate over what to call this new thing happening to people who had had polio was interesting. We formed follow-up subcommittees to try for a uniform approach to research. One of the best outcomes of all this attention and publicity was the mobilization of support groups to gather data and spread the alarm.

Dr. Sass' Chapter 11, entitled "Late Effects," epitomizes the post-polio syndrome story and all of the complications of other traumas and diseases that add to the disability of post-polio syndrome. For many, the new symptoms and awareness reawakened powerful memories. Some are of the sadness of isolation and separation. Some are of embarrassment and chagrin. Many memories recur of kind and interested physicians and therapists, and of family love and sacrifice. I was reminded of the smell of hot packs, of being cut by a cast cutter (after assurances that no one had ever been cut by a cast cutter), and of diversions while isolated that must have annoyed the nurses. Most of us were treated in teaching hospitals and were often used for demonstration. We were usually clad only in little cloth things that barely covered us and our embarrassment. Most of us seem to have been inclined to work hard at what we chose to do in vocational, physical, or recreational activities. Much of this challenge to achieve was associated with a desire to prove capability and capacity in the presence of a physical disability.

The memories jarred loose by reading this book and listening to support group discussions help to define ourselves by understanding better the way we were and by becoming more sensitive to the experiences of others. The stories contain instances of grimness and humor, of courage and fear, of optimism and sadness, of coping and denial. This carefully-put-together book is a service to society as a history of a time and of a disease with broad ramifications and implications. To individuals with polio residuals and/or post-polio syndrome and their families, the book serves as a collective memoir. To those health workers, scientists, and volunteers who participated in the battles against this frightening and often devastating disease, the book can function as recognition for a job well done. The miracle behind so many of the individual histories was the recovery that was made possible by the strange, wide-ranging regrowth of nerve fibers to paralyzed muscles and the fact that this unnatural mechanism served us so well and for so long. Dr. Sass and his co-workers should be congratulated and applauded for their excellent job in creating *Polio's Legacy: An Oral History*. This type of issue-specific oral history should serve as a model for future historians in recording the battles by society and individuals against formidable diseases and events.

Richard Owen, M.D.

PREFACE

I was diagnosed with polio during the first week of June, 1953. Though that event was to powerfully affect the rest of my life, I remember very little of it. I was, after all, only six years old and very ill. I do remember being carried into the hospital, having a spinal tap to confirm the diagnosis, and either dreaming or hallucinating that a flock of angels was having a picnic on the empty bed across the double room where I spent the first night of my hospitalization. Though I was there for the better part of the month, I remember only little snippets of that June. Things like getting *six* shots a day and not being able to stand without holding onto the bed stick in my mind. I also have a vivid image of the heavy, double, French-type doors that separated the polio ward from the rest of the hospital. I was home for the Fourth of July and have a clear recollection of lying on a lounge chair and setting off sparklers.

From there on my memory improves. Even if I wanted to, I couldn't forget the five years I spent in a snug-fitting, metal-and-leather back brace and the three subsequent years I was encased from my hips to my armpits in plaster of Paris. I'm, of course, reminded of my two back surgeries every time I take off my shirt. And some of my most vivid childhood memories involve being stared at, teased, pitied, or just plain avoided by other children and even many adults. I also clearly recall the look on my parents' faces when our insurance agent told them that no more of my polio-related medical bills would be covered.

Today when people ask me why I limp or don't stand straight and I tell them that I had polio as a child, they often give me a blank look. People only a few years younger than I am will sometimes think that polio is a progressive disease or, believing it to be hereditary, will ask if any of my children are affected. A neighbor in her early 30's once asked me if my parents had practiced some sort of strange religion. She must have surmised by the look on my face that I didn't understand the question, so she added, "You know, not to let them vaccinate you." To her, and most others her age, there had always been a polio vaccine. Even people who are older often act surprised that I had polio. Polio is such a distant memory for them that they either had forgotten about it, or they simply no longer associate conditions like mine with the aftereffects of polio. Even most physicians don't know much about polio. And why should they? After all, there hasn't been a major polio outbreak in the United States for over 30 years, and the United Nations reports that polio has been "totally eradicated from the Western Hemisphere" (Report, 1993).

Perhaps that's why I believe a book like this is necessary. It's sort of like the reason the man gave for climbing the mountain - "Because it was there." Well, these stories are also there, but they won't be much longer. Polio survivors are an endangered species. The approximately 400,000 aging polio survivors living in the U.S. are sort of like Edsels; there won't be any more like us, and no one will mourn that fact. When we are gone, so are our stories. And the loss would be more than ours, for these stories tell us much about coping, the resiliency of the human spirit, and living a good life in spite of adversity. From a more academic perspective, documenting the life stories of polio survivors may give us information of pertinence to those with other disabling conditions. As Margaret Campbell noted in describing her Later Life Effects Study, "Developing a better understanding of the late effects of polio can serve as an important prototype for understanding the secondary complications associated with other long-term physical disabilities, such as cerebral palsy, rheumatoid arthritis, and spinal cord injury" (Cited in Headley, 1995, p. 7).

Actually, when I first conceived of this project three years ago, I had neither an academic nor even a non-academic agenda in mind. Rather, I was thinking only about the stories we polio survivors might be able to tell. I was on vacation with my family, and to pass the time in the airport and during our flight, I began reading a book titled *Everything We Had* (Santoli, 1981), an oral history of the Vietnam war. I couldn't put the book down. The first-hand accounts of these men's and women's experiences in Vietnam were fascinating.

Then it occurred to me. Polio survivors also have stories to tell. We received no purple hearts or even belated recognition for the wounds we received. Nevertheless, we have stories about them, stories that need to be told. As I learned through this study, some of the stories are heartbreaking, others inspiring; a few are even funny. Many of the stories also give us a window to a different time, a time when most children lived in traditional, two-parent families, when there was more of a sense of community, and people took care of their own. But it was also a time when there was no concern for handicapped rights or accessibility, a time before political correctness, when a person with a physical disability was just a "cripple."

When I started work on this project, I thought it would be a relatively easy task. All I had to do was interview some polio survivors, transcribe their stories, and compile them for publication. Well, to some extent that is all there was to it, but it's a more difficult and time-consuming task than it appears. First, there was the problem of finding a number of polio survivors willing to share their stories. The people at Sister Kenny Institute in Minneapolis were very helpful in that regard. They put a description of my planned project in their newsletter and asked any interested polio survivors to contact me. Sister Kenny Institute also provided this same project description to area newspapers, many of which ran it. From these notices, I received many letters and phone calls, actually too many to interview in a timely manner by myself. For that reason, I enlisted the aid of two colleagues, Dr. Anthony Sorem, Associate Professor of Psychology, and Dr. George Gottfried, Associate Professor of Social Work, who helped with the interviewing.

Getting those we interviewed to tell their stories was not a problem. We got the sense that these people had all these stories bottled up inside them just waiting to be told. For the most part, however, these are not the sorts of stories that spouses, friends, or one's children want to hear. For that reason, many of the stories had not been told before or at least had not been told for many years.

In all, we interviewed and/or corresponded with over 40 individuals. Though they resided in a variety of states at the time of their acute illness, most are currently living in the upper midwest. The interviews were tape recorded, then transcribed and edited. Both of these latter tasks were also more difficult than I anticipated. Editing was done just for the sake of readability. In no case was the content of an interview intentionally altered.

The individuals whose stories are included in this book represent varying types and degrees of disability and had a wide range of polio-related experiences. However, we make no claim that they are representative of the entire population of polio survivors.

The interviews were generally conducted in the homes of the interviewees. A standard set of questions was used. These questions asked the individuals to describe their recollections of the day they were diagnosed with polio; their initial stay in the hospital; the types of therapy, surgeries, and other treatment they received; the impact of polio on their childhood, their family, their relationships, and their adulthood; and finally, to describe any post-polio symptoms they had experienced. In addition to the clinical and medical information, we asked those we interviewed to tell us their best polio-related stories. Most obliged.

The book begins with a chapter that provides information about polio. It describes the disease, its current status, history, and some of the mysteries that still surround it. Stories of 35 of those we interviewed follow. These stories are organized into 10 thematic chapters based on common elements in the life experiences of our interviewees. The book ends with an attempt to draw some conclusions from the interviews, an attempt to make some sense of polio's legacy, if that's possible. For, if nothing else, these interviews have taught us that the possible effects of polio on one's life are almost infinite.

Edmund Sass, Ed.D.

Acknowledgements

This book could not have become a reality without the help of many individuals and organizations. We express sincere gratitude to those who have offered both assistance and support over the three and one-half years that it took to complete this project.

For their assistance in helping us locate a sample of polio survivors who would be willing to share their stories, we are very grateful to the Sister Kenny Institute. Without their help, this project never would have gotten off the ground.

Dr. Richard Owen's help with this project has been extraordinary. Not only did he write the book's "Foreword" and allow us to include his polio story, but he also read the initial draft to help insure its medical accuracy. Since he is mentioned by so many of our interviewees, this book is as much his as it is ours.

The encouragement, support, and helpful information offered by Joan Headly of the International Polio Network and the Gazette International Networking Institute (GINI) is greatly appreciated. We polio survivors are fortunate to have an organization such as GINI working on our behalf.

Many individuals helped with the editing of this document. These include Scott Buzard, S. Ann Marie Biermaier, Ed.D.; Richard Wielkiewicz, Ph.D.; David Leitzman, Ed.D.; and James Berry, Ph.D. Because of his training as a neurochemist, Dr. Berry was particularly helpful in assuring the accuracy of the medical and technical aspects of the book.

The work done by Maryjean Opitz in formatting, editing, and typing was invaluable. Without her help, and most of all her patience and kindness, this work never would have been completed.

Finally, I would like to offer my personal gratitude to Nancy Hutchison, M.D. of the Sister Kenny Institute. Without her remarkable medical skill, my own post-polio problems would have prevented me from spending the countless hours at my word processor that a project like this requires.

Chapter 1

Polio: Its Definition, History, Current Status, and Late Effects

Polio, or more properly, poliomyelitis, was one of the most feared and most studied diseases of the first half of the 20th century. Though the Salk and later the Sabin vaccines have essentially eliminated the disease in developed countries, many mysteries and enigmas regarding polio remain. This is probably due to the fact that as polio epidemics ended in North America and Europe, research on the disease and its treatment also came to an abrupt halt. Thus, as LaForce (1983) noted, knowledge about the epidemiology and pathology of polio is essentially frozen at a mid-1950's level.

In this chapter, I will define the disease of polio and explore some of the mysteries that still surround it. I will also present a brief account of the history of the disease and will end the chapter by examining the post-polio syndrome (or sequelae), a mystery of urgent concern for those of us living with polio's late effects.

What is Poliomyelitis?

According to Taber (1970), poliomyelitis is an "inflammation of the gray matter of the spinal cord" (p. P-77). Though the word sounds impressive, it was formed simply by putting together the Greek words describing the site of the disease - *polios* meaning gray, *myelos* meaning marrow - and adding the English suffix *itis*, meaning inflammation. It has gone by many names including infantile paralysis, Heine-Medin's disease, debility of the lower extremities,

and spinal paralytic paralysis.   In common usage, the term
poliomyelitis is abbreviated to *polio*.

Polio is caused by a virus which results in an acute infection.
However, contrary to what is commonly believed, the virus does *not*
typically result in paralysis.   Actually, the majority of infected
individuals experienced only mild respiratory or gastrointestinal
symptoms, often accompanied by fever, headache, and muscle
stiffness. These symptoms lasted only a few days, and many had
such mild cases that they did not even realize they were ill.
Therefore, they continued on with their daily routines, attending
school and work, and exposing many others to the polio virus. This
helps to explain the many reports by our interviewees that they were
the only ones in their family, neighborhood, or community to "have
had polio." In actuality, there could have been many people with
whom they came into contact who had the *minor* illness, as the non-
paralytic form of polio is often called.

Only in a small minority of cases did the virus penetrate the central
nervous system, causing the major illness, or "true polio" as it came
to be known. In these cases, neurons (nerve cells) in the anterior
horns of the spinal cord and the lower brain were affected, resulting
in "tightness in the neck, back, and hamstring muscles as well as
varying degrees of muscle weakness, as paralysis sets in" (Owen,
1990, p. 211). Though there was never a "cure" for polio, most
patients experienced improvement in muscle strength and control after
the acute infection subsided. In some cases, however, motor neurons
were left severely damaged or completely destroyed, resulting in
permanent weakness or paralysis, most commonly to the lower
extremities (Headly, 1995).

There are actually three separate strains or immunologic types of
the disease: Type I (Brunhide), Type II (Lansing), and Type III
(Leon). Most epidemics, at least in the United States, were the result
of the Type I virus (Nathanson and Martin, 1979).

The means by which the polio virus reaches the central nervous
system is not definitely known (Taber, 1970).   However, it is
interesting to note that relatively recent research conducted with third-
world populations suggests that when those experiencing acute polio
are given injections such as DPT immunizations, antibiotics,
antimalarials, or antipyretics, the injected limb develops paralysis
within one week (LaForce, 1983).

Though this connection between injections and paralysis has
repeatedly been demonstrated, "the mechanism by which this

phenomenon occurs is not well understood. (However) the best evidence to date suggests the trauma initiates a reflex dilation of blood vessels at the corresponding spinal cord level and facilitates entry of the virus" (LaForce, 1983, p. 30). Since excessive muscle strain and fatigue have been reported to be predisposing factors to paralytic polio, it could well be that the same sort of mechanism occurs with motor neurons controlling those muscles that were overworked.

Other factors thought to predispose individuals to the major paralytic disease were pregnancy, tonsillectomy, and other nose and throat procedures. Why these conditions were likely to increase the risk of the disease entering the central nervous system remains unknown.

There is still some mystery surrounding the exact mechanism by which polio is transmitted. As Smith (1990) wrote in her history of the development of the Salk vaccine, "Nobody has ever completely settled the question of how polio is spread, though the best evidence suggests the virus is excreted in the stool and passed through hand-to-hand contact..." (p. 36).

This belief that the polio virus is spread by contact with the feces of an already infected person has been offered as an explanation for the increased incidence of polio in developed countries such as the United States during the 20th century. According to this theory, before the advent of modern sewage treatment plants and other improvements in public sanitation, virtually all individuals came into contact with the polio virus early in their lives when they were at least partially protected by maternal antibodies. Thus, they developed a mild, non-paralytic case, probably during infancy, which provided them with lifelong immunity. However, with better sanitation, both these early infections as well as the likelihood of receiving antibody protection decreased, resulting in greater susceptibility and possible paralysis. Thus, in the words of Smith:

> Put simply, paralytic polio was an inadvertent by-product of modern sanitary conditions. When people were no longer in contact with the open sewers and privies that had once exposed them to the polio virus in very early infancy when paralysis rarely occurs, the disease changed from an endemic condition so mild that no one knew of its existence to a seemingly new epidemic threat of mysterious origins and terrifyingly unknown scope (p. 35).

This central theory regarding the spread of polio is supported, at least to some extent, by experiences in third-world countries. During World War II, for instance, U.S. and British troops stationed in undeveloped countries were much more likely to contract polio than native peoples, who apparently had already developed immunity (Paul, 1971). Even in the 1970's, when individuals from developed countries came into contact with those from a country without a modern sanitation system, the incidence of paralytic polio was about 20 times greater for those from the developed country (Nathanson and Martin, 1979).

The above explanation for the transmission of polio is generally accepted and seems quite logical. However, the incidence of the disease in the United States during the epidemic years was very irregular, not only from year to year, but from area to area, apparently showing no relation to improvements in sewage treatment. The actual reason for this variation remains another of the polio mysteries. However, it has been suggested that this variability was possibly due to increased virulence of certain virus strains or the presence of environmental conditions that enhanced the disease's transmission (Nathanson and Martin, 1979).

Regarding the second factor of environmental conditions, it is well documented that polio was primarily a disease of the summer months. Readers old enough to recall the epidemic years of the 1940's and 50's probably have vivid recollections of community swimming pools and other public areas being closed during the "dog days" of July and August. Perhaps this was an appropriate precaution. The disease occurred 35 times more frequently in August than in April (the month of lowest incidence). Though no one really knows why this was the case, it does not appear that seasonal variation in interpersonal contacts is a sufficient explanation. Rather, it is more likely that warm, moist weather favored transmission of the disease, as Bradshaw (1989) and others have noted. This is, however, just a hypothesis. The actual reason for the seemingly random appearance of polio epidemics remains a mystery to this day. Since the disease is all but dead, it seems unlikely that all of polio's mysteries will ever be solved.

Polio's many complexities became all too apparent to those involved in the search for ways to treat and prevent it. The history of that search is described in the next section of this chapter.

A Polio Chronology

Since polio is the only common disease which results in the paralysis of a previously healthy child, John Paul (1971), from whose detailed history much of the information in this chronology was drawn, had anticipated that its history should be relatively easy to trace. He later concluded, however, that this is not the case. Though there are many descriptions of lame and crippled children in the *Bible* and other early writings, the descriptions are typically too brief to be undeniably identified as polio-related.

Still, there is a general consensus that cases of polio, if not sporadic epidemics, pre-date recorded history. As evidence of the early existence of poliomyelitis, Paul and other writers offer an Egyptian stele (stone carving) dating between 1580 and 1350 B.C. that shows a young man with an atrophied leg, which looks very much like a limb deformity caused by polio.

It was not until the late 1700's, however, that the existence of polio was described with any degree of certainty. After numerous 18th century outbreaks, a British physician named Michael Underwood provided the first clinical description, referring to polio as "debility of the lower extremities" (Paul, 1971, p. 23).

Little was written about polio in the early part of the 19th century until the appearance of Jacob Heine's work. A German physician, Heine published a 78-page monograph in 1840 which not only described the clinical features of the disease, but also noted that its symptoms suggested the involvement of the spinal cord. Yet, the limited medical knowledge of the time and the sub-microscopic nature of the polio virus kept Heine and others from understanding the contagious nature of the disease. Even with the relatively large outbreaks of polio that occurred in Europe during the second half of the 19th century, physicians speculated causes such as teething, stomach upset, and trauma (Paul, 1971).

The first major polio epidemic reported in the United States occurred in Vermont during the summer of 1894. It consisted of 132 total cases, including some adults. Again, causation was attributed to such factors as "overheating, chilling, trauma, fatigue, and such illnesses as typhoid fever, whooping cough, and pneumonia" (Paul, 1971, p. 85).

Not until 1908 was the actual polio virus identified by two Austrian physicians, Karl Landsteiner and E. Popper. Following their discovery, polio became a reportable disease entity, and the state of

Massachusetts began counting polio cases in 1909 (Bradshaw, 1989).

It was during that same year that American physician Simon Flexner successfully induced polio infection in monkeys. This allowed for increased research opportunities as well as unwarranted optimism concerning a "polio cure." However, this optimism quickly subsided, and by 1913 the complexities of prevention and treatment had become apparent (Paul, 1971).

The year 1916 saw a large outbreak of polio in the United States. Though the total number of affected individuals is unknown, over 9000 cases were reported in New York City alone. Attempts at controlling the disease largely involved the use of isolation and quarantine. Though these measures proved ineffective, quarantines during polio outbreaks were continued for many decades.

The 1920's saw the development and first use of the infamous "iron lung," a metal coffin-like contraption that aided respiration, but imprisoned those polio patients who needed it, in some cases for life. However, most polio-related research during this decade centered on the "therapeutic use of convalescent serum" to treat acute polio patients (Paul, 1971). This "serum" was made from the blood of monkeys and humans who had recently recovered from polio and was administered by injection. Based on the results of several small, poorly-designed research studies, as well as the fact that a similar approach had apparently been successful in treating meningitis, some physicians were convinced that this "treatment" could prevent paralysis. Even serum from "hyperimmunized" horses was tried. Hopes for the effectiveness of convalescent serums ran high until the early 1930's when results of several relatively well-conducted field trials yielded discouraging results. As Paul noted:

> The demise of serum therapy after so many years of crude trials on which claims of its value had been made by so many physicians, a number of whom were acknowledged authorities and occupied high places in the medical hierarchy, must have been a bitter pill to swallow - if such a metaphor is appropriate (p. 198).

So, after about two decades of hope, this form of treatment was abandoned. Like so many other "polio treatments," the only positive thing that could be said for serum's use was that at least it wasn't harmful.

With medical research during this decade being essentially a bust, probably the most important polio-related event of the 1920's had nothing to do with medical advances. Rather, it was the fact that Franklin Delano Roosevelt was struck with the disease in 1921. Not a typical polio patient by any means, FDR was 39 years of age at the time and had been his party's vice presidential candidate in 1920.

His misfortune proved to be a stroke of luck, not only for polio victims, but for those with other disabilities as well. FDR's crippling illness was to have a major impact on public perceptions of the handicapped, which tended to be very negative. As Longmore (1987) stated, individuals with physical handicaps were typically, "kept at home, out of sight, in back bedrooms by families who felt a mixture of embarrassment and shame about their presence" (p. 359). Even those in the medical profession tended to look on "cripples" with disdain. "Declared an influential orthopedic text in 1911: a failure in the moral training of a cripple means the evolution of an individual detestable in character, a menace and a burden to the community, who is only apt to graduate into the mendicant and criminal classes" (Longmore, 1987, p. 359). Whether this view was due to a belief that "cripples" were somehow being punished by God for their sins is difficult to surmise, but because of these attitudes it is not surprising that physically disabled children were likely to be barred from attending public schools. Though these negative attitudes and tendencies toward devaluation were well ingrained, a careful strategy of public imagemaking of FDR as being heroically triumphant in spite of his physical limitations contributed to a limited form of acceptance for those with handicaps, at least as long as they didn't complain and continued their "cheerful striving toward normalization" (Longmore, 1987, p. 361).

At least as important as FDR's impact on attitudes towards and treatment of the handicapped was the effect of his prestige and his family's wealth on advances in the treatment and prevention of polio. Much of the story of his impact on the battle against the disease is tied to Warm Springs, Georgia, a place he visited in October, 1924 because of reports that the waters there could somehow "cure" paralysis. A dilapidated resort when he first visited, Roosevelt purchased it 18 months later. He soon renovated and expanded it. Warm Springs became his second home, and it soon became a magnet for polio survivors and others with physical handicaps.

In 1926, the Warm Springs Foundation was started. It was eventually to become the National Foundation for Infantile Paralysis. Under the direction of FDR's law partner, D. Basil O'Connor, this non-profit foundation became national in scope. It not only led the way in galvanizing public interest in polio, but also played a crucial role in raising millions of dollars for the treatment of polio patients and polio-related research.

The decade of the 1930's saw an increase in the frequency and magnitude of polio outbreaks in the United States. Most notable among the epidemics was one that occurred in Los Angeles during the summer of 1934. Nearly 2500 polio cases were treated from May through November of that year at Los Angeles County General Hospital alone. The city was panic-stricken with the appearance of "50 new cases a day" (Paul, 1971, p. 221).

However, the 1930's were also years of medical advances and much hope. It was during this decade the discovery was made that there were at least two separate strains of polio virus. (It was later determined that there were three strains.) Even more noteworthy, though, were the attempts by two physicians to develop a polio vaccine. These efforts culminated in 1935 with field trials for vaccines developed by Maurice Brodie and John Kollmer. Using what Paul referred to as "kitchen chemistry" (p. 258), the two hurried their "vaccines" into readiness, each fearing the other would succeed first. Brodie concocted his from an emulsion of the ground-up spinal cords of infected monkeys. He attempted to deactivate the virus by exposing it to formalin (a formaldehyde mixture). This formalin-inactivated concoction was first tried with 20 monkeys, then with 3000 children. Though it is unclear exactly what occurred, "something went wrong and Brodie's vaccine was never used again" (Paul, 1971, p. 256).

Kollmer's attempt at developing a vaccine was based on a slightly different premise. His idea was to use live, but slightly weakened (attenuated) virus, again taken from the spinal cords of infected monkeys. The virus was attenuated by mixing it with various chemicals and refrigerating it for 14 days. Paul called the result a "veritable witches' brew" (p. 258). After trying his "vaccine" on a few monkeys, himself, his children, and 22 others, Kollmer was optimistic enough to distribute thousands of doses to physicians across the country. Unfortunately, the vaccine was not only ineffective, but was blamed for causing many cases of polio, some of which were fatal. In his remarks at a meeting of the Southern Branch of the American Public Health Association held in 1935, Kollmer is reported to have said, "Gentlemen, this is one time I wish the floor would open up and swallow me" (Paul, 1971, p. 260).

In spite of his failed attempts at vaccine development, Kollmer apparently managed to pick up the pieces and go on to a successful, if not distinguished, research career. This was not the case for Brodie. Unable to find an important research position, he died shortly after accepting a minor position in Michigan. "It is alleged that he took his own life" (Paul, 1971, p. 261). Thus, tragically, he did not live to see Salk's successful development of a polio vaccine based on his concept of using formalin-inactivated virus. Even more tragically for the hundreds of thousands who contracted polio in the 1940's and 50's, the 1935 fiasco made the scientific community so gun shy that polio vaccine trials on human subjects were not attempted again for nearly 20 years.

As most of the developed world became embroiled in the Second World War, the first half of the decade of the 1940's saw few new polio-related developments. One important exception to this was the arrival in the United States of Sister Elizabeth Kenny and her then unorthodox approach to polio treatment.

Not a nun, Elizabeth Kenny was a former Australian army nurse. The title "Sister" was a reference to her military rank as chief nurse, and had no religious connection. In her work with Australian polio patients, Sister Kenny had developed a treatment procedure that involved massage, exercises, and wrapping affected limbs with hot, moist compresses to reduce muscle spasms and the resultant pain. She also stressed the importance of psychotherapy in treatment, insisting children had to be "willed to move paralyzed limbs" (Willis, 1979, p. 32). This approach was totally contrary to the accepted medical treatment of the time which typically involved long-term splinting and casting to immobilize the limbs, combined with prolonged bed rest. Unfortunately for the many who received it, this standard practice of immobilization did more harm than good, causing only atrophy and inflexibility in already weakened limbs.

After years of meeting with resistance from the Australian medical establishment, in 1940 the 53-year-old Kenny came to the United States to promote her ideas. In his monograph for the Hennepin County Historical Society, Don Albertson (1978) wrote that she arrived first in California where she was virtually ignored by the medical community. After getting a similarly cool reception in New York from D. Basil O'Connor, then chairman of the National Foundation for Infantile Paralysis, Kenny decided to return to Australia. However, because she had letters of introduction to physicians in Chicago and at the Mayo Clinic in Rochester,

Minnesota, she decided to stop in those two cities before leaving for home.

Fortunately, she found the people in the Midwest at least friendlier, if not necessarily enthusiastic about her ideas. Albertson quoted Kenny as remarking, "The whole city of Rochester, in fact, seemed to exude friendliness" (p. 2). She also found some physicians in Rochester who were at least willing to listen to her and gave the first presentation in the United States regarding her procedures to members of the Mayo Clinic staff. Though impressed with her ideas, there were no acute polio patients being treated at Mayo at that time. Therefore, Kenny was referred to Doctors Wallace Cole and Miland Knapp in Minneapolis, where there were many acute cases.

Cole and Knapp arranged for her to work with some of their more severe cases, including Robert Gurney, who was interviewed for this book. Since she achieved some success with these patients, other physicians soon invited her to work with their patients. According to Albertson, "Each week saw more cases showing benefits of her techniques, and soon it became necessary to find facilities to handle the cases that were brought to her" (p. 5).

Before long, she had an entire ward at Minneapolis General Hospital (now Hennepin General) set up for her work, and a year later additional space was provided at the University of Minnesota Hospital. Shortly thereafter, the first Sister Kenny Institute opened on December 17, 1942. The Sister Elizabeth Kenny Foundation was formed in 1943 to support both her work with polio patients and to further the teaching of her methods.

Her methods remained controversial, however, and a report of a special American Medical Association committee first published in 1944 was very critical of the Kenny approach (Committee, 1969). The National Foundation never embraced her ideas and finally gave them only a grudging endorsement, acknowledging that the "treatment had some basis in fact" (Paul, 1971, p. 342). Nevertheless, by the mid-1940's, the Kenny method had become pretty much the standard treatment for polio patients in the United States. Though there does not appear to be scientific research to substantiate any long-term benefits of the method, it was certainly preferable to the traditional approach of immobilization.

Elizabeth Kenny died in 1952, but her followers continued her work. In fact, the Sister Kenny Institute is still in existence and continues to provide services to disabled persons. Though polio is no longer its primary mission, the Institute offers evaluation and treatment for post-polio patients and is a leader in research and dissemination of information on the late effects of polio.

Other than Sister Kenny's impact on the treatment of those with paralytic polio, the early 1940's saw little other progress in either prevention or treatment. Most of the best medical researchers were either in the military or working on military-related projects. Therefore, their civilian research interests were put on the back burner. However, some, including Jonas Salk, would later apply the knowledge they gained from research conducted for the military to their work on polio.

Other polio-related information gained during World War II was learned the hard way. Experiences of Allied military troops further confirmed adult susceptibility to polio. This was particularly the case when they were stationed in locations with primitive sanitation systems. U.S. and British personnel in Africa, the Middle East, and the Philippines were hit particularly hard. With the occurrence of large epidemics of polio in the U.S. immediately after the war (an average of more than 20,000 cases a year during the period 1945-49), it was speculated by some that service personnel may have "brought the virus home with them" (Smith, 1990, p. 86).

The combination of large scale post-war polio epidemics and the discharge of medical researchers from their military obligations resulted in renewed interest in polio research. Most of this research now centered on vaccine development. Though Jonas Salk would eventually develop the first effective vaccine, he was a newcomer to the field of polio research. In fact, in her book detailing the story of the vaccine's development, Jane Smith has stated that Salk actually became involved in polio research only as a means of obtaining funding for his new laboratory in Pittsburgh.

This laboratory, funded by the Sarah Mellon Scientific Foundation as an attempt to put Pittsburgh on the medical map, opened shop in 1947. As one of its first projects, Salk's facility was one of four laboratories awarded research grants for the polio virus-typing project, which began in 1948. Though it was long suspected that there were three separate antigenic types of polio virus, this would need to be definitely known so that a vaccine could provide protection against all viral strains. This project was seen by Salk as "a dull but dependable investment that would provide a regular dividend of money for his lab..." (Smith, 1990, p. 117). Though Salk had not previously been involved in polio research, his participation in the Armed Forces Epidemiological Board, which worked on the development of influenza vaccines during the war, provided him with invaluable experience for both virus typing and, eventually, polio vaccine development (Paul, 1971).

According to Smith, Salk's newness to the study of the polio virus may actually have benefitted him. Since he had no involvement in an ongoing polio research program, he started out fresh, without preconceived notions. Perhaps this is why he was the only polio researcher to use the tissue-culture method of cultivating and working with the polio virus that had recently been developed by John Enders and others at Harvard University. Other researchers, including Albert Sabin, who would later develop the oral polio vaccine, continued to do their work with monkeys infected with the polio virus, a more difficult and time-consuming process.

Salk's work on the influenza virus during the war gave him another advantage over others studying the polio virus. In his attempts at developing an influenza vaccine, he had worked with "killed virus." Therefore, it was only natural for him to use this same approach to developing a polio vaccine. Sabin and the others who were already involved in polio vaccine development were using live, attenuated (weakened) virus, again a more difficult task.

Resurrecting the idea of using formalin-inactivated (killed) virus tried by Brodie in his failed work of the 1930's, by 1950, Salk and his cohorts were already leading the way in developing a polio vaccine. According to a *Time Magazine* article which appeared in 1953 ("Vaccine"), Salk added mineral water to his formaldehyde-treated virus as a means of holding the virus in the body long enough to enhance the formation of antibodies, just as mineral oils were added to hold penicillin in the system.

By 1952, early versions of his vaccine had already proven successful with small samples of patients at the Watson Home for Crippled Children and the Polk State School, a Pennsylvania facility for the mentally retarded (Paul, 1971; Smith, 1990). Salk reported the results of these promising, albeit small-scale, studies to the National Foundation's Committee on Polio Vaccination in January, 1953. Perhaps because the country had just experienced the worst polio epidemic in history (about 58,000 cases in 1952), the committee went against the urgings of Sabin and others and decided to back Salk's work. Massive national field trials, the magnitude of which were never seen before *or* since, were organized a year later to test the vaccine's effectiveness.

According to Mierer (1972), nearly 2 million children participated in the 1954 field trials at a cost of about 5 million dollars. (One can only guess what the cost would be today!) Mierer states that these large numbers were necessary because of the "relatively low incidence of the disease and its great variability from place to place and time to time..." (pp. 5 and 6).

There was some disagreement in the scientific community regarding exactly how the field trials should be conducted. One plan which was backed by the National Foundation proposed to offer vaccination to second graders at participating schools and compare them to non-vaccinated first and third graders in the same schools (an "observed-control approach"). This plan was criticized by some scientists, however, because the physicians eventually charged with making the polio diagnosis would know whether or not a child had been vaccinated. Thus, their judgement could be biased. Additionally, since only children whose parents had volunteered their participation would be vaccinated, some differences, particularly in socio-economic status, were likely to exist between the vaccinated and non-vaccinated groups.

To overcome these objections, it was proposed that children be randomly assigned to vaccinated or non-vaccinated groups, with those not vaccinated receiving an injection of a saline (salt) solution colored to look exactly like the Salk vaccine. Not the children, their parents, nor even their physicians would know whether a child had been given the real vaccine or the placebo, saline solution. This "placebo-control approach" overcame the arguments of potentially biased results. However, there were objections on ethical grounds as some wondered about the appropriateness of giving children a "fake" vaccine for a feared and potentially deadly disease (Mierer, 1972).

In the end, both approaches were used, and the decision regarding in which study to participate was left to individual departments of health. Eventually, about 750,000 children participated in the placebo-control study, and slightly over a million in the observed-control experiment. Though the placebo-control study was judged more conclusive, results of the two studies were similar. The vaccine was not totally effective in preventing polio, but those vaccinated were less than one-half as likely to contract polio as the non-vaccinated control group. Additionally, in those cases where a vaccinated child was diagnosed with polio, the disease was more likely to be judged as non-paralytic (Mierer, 1972).

News of the successful vaccine trials was released at a formal press conference held in Ann Arbor, Michigan (the site where the research data from the field trials had been gathered and analyzed) on April 12, 1955. It was broadcast on both radio and television. Though some in the scientific community criticized the manner in which the announcement was made as sensationalized, the results were greeted with public euphoria.

> Flushed by the first report that the vaccine had worked, exuberant citizens rushed to ring church bells and fire sirens, shouted, clapped, sang and made every kind of joyous noise they could. City councils and state legislatures postponed their regular business to draft resolutions congratulating Salk for his wonderful achievement (Smith, 1990, p. 319).

Following the public announcement, a nationwide vaccination program was quickly undertaken. Though several pharmaceutical companies were contracted to produce the vaccine, during the first year (1955) only enough could be manufactured to vaccinate about one-third of the roughly 18 million children and adolescents under the age of 20 (Jones, 1993). However, by 1957, ample supplies were already available to vaccinate everyone. Surprisingly, not all chose to have their children vaccinated, and so a large-scale advertising campaign was initiated, including the public vaccination of Elvis Presley (Smith, 1990). In spite of this measure, by 1960 only about 71% of those under the age of 20 were fully vaccinated with another 15% partially vaccinated (Jones, 1993).

In any operation of this magnitude, of course, not everything will go exactly as planned, and the polio vaccination program was no exception. Unfortunately, some of those vaccinated actually developed polio, apparently from the vaccine. It was later learned that some of the lots of vaccine manufactured by Cutter Laboratories of California contained live polio virus. Fortunately, this was the only such incident (Paul, 1971).

Though apparently no study was ever conducted to examine the long-term effectiveness of the Salk vaccine, the statistics dramatically illustrate at least its short-term success. From pre-vaccine highs of about 58,000 cases in 1952 and 35,000 cases in 1953, the rate dropped to about 5600 cases in 1957, the first year after the vaccine was widely available (Jones, 1993).

By 1962, the Salk vaccine was replaced by the Sabin oral vaccine. The effectiveness of this new vaccine had been demonstrated in field trials conducted in 1958 and 1959. Using live, attenuated (weakened) virus, the oral vaccine was not only superior in terms of ease of administration, but also provided longer-lasting immunization (Nathanson, 1982).

With the Salk and later the Sabin vaccines providing a one-two punch, polio was down and out for the count, at least in the United States. In 1964, only 121 cases were reported nationally. Currently, there are typically fewer than 10 new cases per year, but none originates from native, "wild" polio virus. Rather, these cases are either vaccine-related or "imported" (Nathanson, 1982).

There were still about 100,000 cases of polio worldwide during 1993 (Keegan, 1994). However, there has not been a case of polio due to native, wild polio virus in the entire western hemisphere since 1991 (Report, 1993), and if Target 2000, sponsored by Rotary International, is successful, the entire world will be free of polio within the next few years. Polio's legacy remains, however. In 1977, the National Health Interview Survey reported that there were 254,000 persons living in the United States who had been paralyzed by polio (Frick and Bruno, 1986), and the total number of polio survivors in this country may still exceed 400,000. The number worldwide is probably more than 10 million, many of whom must be suffering from polio's late effects.

Polio's Late Effects

With the extermination of the polio virus in the United States, polio became an all-but-forgotten disease. For the most part, those of us who had it learned to cope with whatever residual disabilities the disease had caused. We married, had children, progressed in our careers, and lived essentially ordinary lives. We gave the disease that had so disrupted our childhoods little thought. Whatever damage it had done occurred decades ago, and we thought it would not affect us again. We were wrong. This disease isn't a quitter. Almost as if its ghost had risen to avenge its death, polio slipped back into the news in the early 1980's with reports that many polio survivors were now experiencing new and unexpected symptoms.

Actually, there had been periodic evidence of late polio effects dating back to the 1800's, and it has been suggested that F.D.R. was experiencing these late effects toward the end of his life (Speier, Owen, Knapp, and Canine, 1990). Still, it was thought that these were isolated, atypical cases. In the late 1970's, however, a former polio patient wrote to the *Rehabilitation Gazette*, a newsletter for the disabled, reporting increased muscle weakness. Many other polio survivors responded, describing similar symptoms, and the magnitude of the problem started to become apparent. The national media soon pounced on this phenomenon and began running features on "the crippler's return."

Symptoms most typically reported by those experiencing these late effects are: (1) excessive fatigue and reduced endurance; (2) new joint and muscle pain; (3) progressive muscle weakness, not only in muscles previously affected, but also in muscles apparently unaffected by acute polio; (4) new or increased breathing difficulties, in some cases requiring the use of ventilatory devices; and (5) cold intolerance that contributes to muscle weakness and is accompanied by burning pain (Jones, Speier, Canine, and Owen, 1989). The severity of the symptoms is quite variable, and in some cases individuals may require additional bracing, or may find that they now need canes or a wheelchair. Lifestyle changes may also be necessary (Owen, 1990).

These post-polio symptoms have been given a variety of names including post-poliomyelitis progressive muscular atrophy (PPMA), late effects of acute poliomyelitis, and most commonly, post-polio syndrome. The Post-Polio Research Task Force prefers the term post-polio sequelae, but because post-polio problems tend to be vague and ill-defined, perhaps Dr. David Bodian's suggestion of "things that happen to people who once had polio" is the most appropriate title (Owen and Speier, 1986).

Since no one had predicted that these "things" would happen to polio survivors, physicians typically did not attribute the symptoms to the late effects of polio. Thus, as was the case for some of those whose stories appear in this book, polio patients often experienced frustration and depression due to misdiagnosis (Frick and Bruno, 1986).

Typically the new symptoms begin about 30 years after the acute polio infection. Though the symptoms may be acutely precipitated by illness or injury, usually their onset is gradual. Therefore, it is often difficult for individuals to pinpoint exactly when they started to experience new polio-related problems.

Estimates of the prevalence of post-polio sequelae vary greatly. Owen (1990) reported that surveys provide estimates ranging between 20 and 80%. Figures of 20 to 40% may be more realistic, however. A study conducted by the Mayo Clinic in Rochester, Minnesota found that 22% of their subjects were experiencing new problems (Codd, et al, 1985), and research conducted at Sister Kenny Institute in Minneapolis found new problems reported by 41% (Speier, Owen, Knapp, and Canine, 1990). Though not consistently found in all studies, it appears that those who contracted polio after age 10 are more likely to develop post-polio symptoms (Speier, Owen, Knapp, and Canine, 1987). Additionally, those most impaired at the time of their acute illness and who then experienced the most recovery of function may also be at a greater risk (Headly, 1995).

The cause of post-polio syndrome is another of polio's many enigmas. Though some writers have speculated that it may be due to persistent or recurrent infection with the polio virus (Shariff, Phil, Hentges, and Ciardi, 1991), most researchers have found no evidence of recurrent infection (Owen, 1990; Yarnell, Wice, and Maynard, 1994). Neither is there evidence that these new symptoms are related to multiple sclerosis or amyotrophic lateral sclerosis (ALS or Lou Gehrig's disease). Rather, it is probable that new, polio-related symptoms have multiple causes including muscle imbalances (i.e. extra stress placed on stronger muscles to compensate for weaker ones), overuse/abuse of weakened muscles (weakened muscles already functioning near capacity may be more susceptible to injury), and deconditioning/undertraining (deconditioning of already weakened muscles may result in reduced strength and stamina sufficient to make walking and other basic functions more difficult).

Premature aging of nerve tissue may be another possible cause (Owen, 1990). People normally experience a very gradual decline in nerve cells and in muscle strength after age 50. However, since those who had polio have already lost some nerve cells, they may experience these declines earlier in life. Additionally, new medical conditions that are a typical part of the aging process for all individuals, may be exacerbated by polio's late effects. As Frederick Maynard noted:

> (This) perspective suggests people with a history of polio residual weakness are especially vulnerable to losses in functional capacity as they age because of an increasing statistical probability that they will develop non-polio related medical problems and experience an exaggerated impact on function from them (Yarnell, Weiss, and Maynard, 1994, p. 9).

Related to the theory of premature aging, research reported by Jones, Speier, Canine, and Owen (1989) suggests that a major cause of the late effects of polio may be "failure of terminal axonal sprout function causing defective transmission at the neuromuscular junction" (p. 3255). While this explanation sounds quite complex, what these writers are saying is that some nerve cells (neurons) that survived the acute polio infection sprouted new axons, somewhat like a tree branch sprouts twigs. These sprouted nerve cells then took over the control of muscle fibers that did not have surviving neurons. The sprouted neurons simply may tend to age and wear out more quickly than normal nerve cells. When the sprouted neurons "drop-out," the individual loses function in the muscle fibers they controlled.

Another theory suggests that new muscle weakness may be a function of neural loss due to "failure of reinnervation" (Yarnell, Wice, and Maynard, 1994). Similar to the previous explanation regarding the failure of sprouted neurons, this perspective holds that some of the nerve cells (neurons) of polio survivors that were destroyed during the acute illness grew back, thus "reinnervating" the muscle fibers they controlled. However, these reinnervated nerve cells often have to supply more than their usual share of muscle fibers in order to compensate for neurons that were not reinnervated. "These giant motor neurons appear to be under great metabolic stress from the high rate of use and muscle fiber turnover (from denervation/reinnervation). Thus, they are thought to be fragile and subject to degenerative fragmentation..." (Yarnell, Wice, and Maynard, 1994, p. 5). Therefore, the new weakness experienced by some polio survivors may occur as a result of a slowing or cessation of the reinnervation process. Though all individuals experience a slowing of reinnervation as they age, this may occur sooner because of overuse, and the resultant loss of function may be more severe for polio survivors because the lost motor neurons may have controlled more muscle fibers.

It has also been recently speculated that some post-polio symptoms, particularly increasing fatigue, may be due to irregularities in the arousal center (reticular activating system) of the brain stem, which was affected in some polio patients. Weakened or damaged neurons in the brain stem may be particularly susceptible to underoxygenation when individuals who lack endurance over-exert themselves. Since it has been shown that many polio survivors are type A personalities, prone to driving themselves to exhaustion (Speier, Owen, Jones, and Seizert, 1990), it may be that they are likely to push themselves to the point where this underoxygenation occurs. Additionally, since the reticular activating system of the brainstem is essential in the body's management of stress, some researchers believe "that, at least in some cases, extreme exhaustion and fatigue may be related to a reduced capacity of the reticular system to respond to what otherwise would appear as... typical daily stress" (Yarnell, Wice, and Maynard, 1994, p.8).

Since the causes of post-polio sequelae are not definitely known, it is not surprising that there currently is no "cure." However, there are ways to ease the symptoms. While some cases may require lifestyle adjustments, bracing, or the use of other aids, an effective approach for some appears to be carefully prescribed aerobic exercises that alternate activity and rest. This sort of exercise program has "been shown to increase conditioning, muscle endurance, and oxygen intake without further damaging weakened muscles" (Owen, 1990, p. 2). It has been found that exercising three times per week gives optimal results (Speier, Owen, Jones, and Seizert, 1990).

The use of exercise in treating the late effects of polio is controversial, however. As reported by Young (1988) and others, some researchers believe that although exercise can produce short-term benefits, its impact may be harmful in the long run. Thus, they recommend that polio survivors be cautious and avoid exercising to the point where they experience increased pain, muscle spasms, or excessive fatigue.

Another approach to the treatment of post-polio syndrome involves the use of medications. Recent research has shown that medications such as Mestinon, which is used with myasthenia gravis patients, and Symetral, most often used with Parkinson's patients, may be of some help. Both of these drugs may improve the functioning of damaged or weakened nerve cells (Speier, Owen, Jones, and Seizert, 1990), and medications such as Elavil that are often prescribed to combat depression, can be helpful in the treatment of polio-related chronic fatigue. Prednisone, a steroid often used to treat multiple sclerosis, is also being used with post-polio patients, and The National Institute of Neurological Disorders and Stroke is currently experimenting with the use of nerve growth factor, "a protein that spurs the proliferation of nerve axons" (Elmer-Dewitt, 1994, p. 55). These and possibly other drugs may become increasingly important in treating post-polio problems in the future.

In conclusion, there does not appear to be a definitive answer to treating polio's late effects, but new information is continually being learned. It is important, therefore, for polio survivors to keep abreast of any and all pertinent developments. Perhaps the best recommendation, however, would be to get a thorough evaluation at a facility with experience treating the late effects of polio (such as Sister Kenny Institute). They may not have all the answers, but at least they will be able to provide the best possible advice for those of us dealing with polio's latest, and hopefully last, challenge.

Chapter 2

"She Carried Herself Like a Queen"

Since so many of those we interviewed were treated with the Sister Kenny method, it seems particularly appropriate that the first of the interview chapters focuses on Elizabeth Kenny and her approach to the treatment of polio. Though they deal with much more, Sister Kenny, her method, and the Sister Kenny Institute are at the heart of the three stories that appear in this chapter. In fact, all three of these men met and were treated directly by Elizabeth Kenny.

Bob Gurney, from whose interview the chapter title was taken, was among the very first acute polio patients to be treated by Elizabeth Kenny in 1940 after her arrival in the United States. Dick Owen, a polio survivor who became a physician and eventually Medical Director of Sister Kenny Institute, met Elizabeth Kenny only once. That meeting occurred when Kenny traveled to Indiana to demonstrate and teach her methods to the staff at the Indiana University Hospital. Dick Owen was one of the young polio patients on whom she demonstrated her methods. Dick's story is interesting not only because of his eventual involvement with the Sister Kenny Institute, but also because it provides a clear contrast between the Kenny method and the traditional treatment approach of prolonged splinting and immobilization.

Ray Gullickson, however, had the most prolonged contact with Sister Kenny. Perhaps his story gives the clearest and most detailed picture of what Elizabeth Kenny was like as a person.

Robert Gurney

I was 17 years old in the summer of 1940. At that time I was a pretty good baseball player. I was a catcher and had hopes of eventually playing in the major leagues. However, I came down with polio in August, and that put an end to my baseball career.

The day before I got sick I had caught a whole baseball game. It was kind of hot that day, especially with all that equipment on, so when I got home I took sort of a cool bath. That next morning, which was a Sunday morning, I woke up with a bit of a headache. By the time I got home from church though, I had a terrific headache, and I started to have a backache, down by my tailbone. I took a couple of aspirins and fell asleep. When I got up, the backache was just as bad as the headache. I called my aunt who was a registered nurse, and the only thing she could think of doing right then was for me to lie on the hot water bottle. That was kind of the standard thing to do back in those days, so I got out the hot water bottle and laid down.

My folks were out of town in Chicago at a convention, and when they got home that afternoon, my mom told me I should take a hot bath. Well, I took a pink bath, and I don't know if that had anything to do with me getting polio or not, but I probably shouldn't have done that because I woke up Monday morning, and I couldn't move. By that time, I was completely paralyzed. I couldn't do anything but move my eyes. My folks called our family doctor, and he called an ambulance. When they picked me up, my mother said the pain was so great that I passed out and became unconscious. The doctor told the ambulance attendants to cover my face with a rubber sheet and then to cover me with the outside blanket. My mother asked why, and he said, "Because we don't know if he's contagious, and we don't want to take any chances." So there I was, paralyzed, and they covered me up with a rubber sheet, but I didn't even notice because I was unconscious most of the time. I must have been able to breathe though, because I'm alive!

They took me to St. Luke's Hospital and tapped my spine. They found out what I had, so they didn't put the fluid back in my spine because it was contaminated. They thought that keeping the fluid out might alleviate the pain and maybe some of the crippling, but it didn't help at all. I guess that's the only thing they knew to do back then.

When the doctor came in my room, he asked, "Do you know what infantile paralysis is?" I told him that I didn't, and then he said, "Polio." I'd heard of it, but nothing like that had ever entered my mind. He told me, "Well that's what you've got. You've got polio, and you did a good job of it. You're going to be crippled from the top of your shoulders to down in your toes." He said, "Oh, I can see the pain." But, you know, the funny part is, I never got a shot for pain, and I never got a pill for pain, except the aspirins I took for my headache.

So, I was in the hospital with polio. Something that I've never understood though, if polio was so contagious, how come I was the only one I knew who got it? I was the only one in the whole darned block. In fact, I played ball with about twenty kids the day before, and I was the only one who got it. I guess that was just my luck.

I ended up staying at St. Luke's Hospital for only two, maybe three days. The bed was tilted so my head was down on the floor the whole time I was there because they had tapped my spine. The room I was in wasn't like a regular hospital room. It was really small, and it had a lot of junk in it. I thought it was a cloak room or a storage room or something like that.

They didn't have a contagion ward at St. Luke's, so that's why they transferred me over to Anchor Hospital where they did have a contagion floor. That hospital (Anchor) isn't in existence anymore. They tore it down. Anyway, they took me over to old Anchor, and they did the same thing again. They put me on the stretcher and covered me up with the rubber sheet. They had the old-time ambulances back then, and you'd lay on the rubber sheet so if you were drunk or whatever there was a rubber sheet under you, and they would fold the rubber sheet over you, including your face, if they wanted. Then they'd put the white sheet over that. If you were paralyzed like I was, you couldn't get it off.

When I got over to Anchor Hospital, I couldn't move anything. My hands were at my sides, and that was it. The doctor would come by every morning and give me a shot of vitamin B 1, the "sunshine vitamin." Like he said, "We don't know if it's going to help, but we know damn well it isn't going to do any harm!"

After I was at Anchor for a few days, they called up my folks from the hospital, or maybe they called my family doctor; I'm not sure, and they told them about Sister Kenny. She had just come to Minneapolis. They said they didn't know if she could help, but I was so completely paralyzed that if I didn't get some kind of help I was going to die. So she certainly couldn't do me any harm. Though I didn't know it yet, I was going to be one of her first patients here.

I don't remember the exact date, but I was lying there, and my mom walked in and said, "I've got somebody here who may be able to help you. This is Sister Elizabeth Kenny." Of course, when she said sister, I was thinking, "What's going on here." But she was standing on the left side of the bed, and she looked down at me and said, "No Bobby, my name is Elizabeth Kenny. The 'sister' means that I am a registered nurse from the Australian Army. That's our title." I looked up at her, and I remember thinking, "Wow, what a big woman." She must have been about six foot one and weighed close to 200, 205, maybe 210 pounds. So she was one big woman, and oh man! She carried herself like a queen. Her size sure didn't bother her at all.

She looked me right in the eye and said, "I'm here to try to help you. But, before I can help you, I've got to hurt you." Well, what could I say? So, she reached across the bed, grabbed my hand, and started shaking it. Then she said, "Now, we'll get started." So she lifted up my left leg and started trying to find out how good or bad it was, and I was damned if I was going to let anybody know how badly it hurt. I wasn't going to yell, but the next thing I knew, I was crying from the pain. She noticed that, so she put down my left leg, but then she started on my right leg, and a few more tears came. Finally, she let go of my right leg and said, "We won't do anything with your arms right now; I'll come back later this afternoon."

She came back that afternoon and was fooling around with my fingers and hands and arms. Then she said to the nurses, "Do you have any old blankets, completely wool blankets?" The nurses told her that they had plenty of them, and so Sister Kenny said, "All right, get me one, and bring me a pair of scissors." So she showed the nurses how to cut strips out of the blankets to fit the arms and legs, and then she said, "We'll need some hot water; we're going to put the blanket in it, and then we have to wring it dry." Well, they've got plenty of hot water at a hospital, but they didn't have any way to get the blankets dry enough. So my mother brought in this little hand wringer, and they put it on the side of the tub that they put the hot water in. They put the pieces of blanket in the hot water; then they wrung them out, and wrapped me up in them. But they didn't have any pieces of plastic to put over the blankets like they should have, so they took out that good old rubber sheet again and covered me up all the way from my toes to under my chin.

They changed the hot packs every half an hour or 45 minutes the first couple of days. And oh man, within about two hours, I didn't have any pain. So from then on, the pain was gone, but I sure didn't like that rubber sheet!

After only a couple of days of the hot packs, my muscles started to relax. Up until then, my muscles were as tight as the strings in a tennis racket. When your muscles are that tight, you can't move anything. I was trying like the dickens to get something to move, but nothing would. And the pain, it's like you had a cramp, but multiply that pain 100 times.

A few days later, my doctor came in, and he had leg splints and arm splints. He put them on me and said, "These will help you." I asked how they could help, and he said, "Well, that's all we know to do." I asked about Sister Kenny, and he told me, "They said I should work with her, but you're my patient, so I'm going to do what I think is right." Of course, I couldn't blame him for that, but when Sister Kenny came back that afternoon, she just stood there and took a look. Then she said to the head floor nurse, "Get me a pair of scissors," and she cut off those splints and threw them on the floor in the corner of the room. And then she said, "You don't need these; who gave them to you?" I told her that my doctor did, and she just smiled and said, "Well, he's just a young doctor; I'll have a talk with him." And that was the last I saw of those splints.

All this time my mom had been picking up Sister Kenny in Minneapolis and driving her to Anchor Hospital in St. Paul to see me. But after about 10 days, my mom came in and told me that Sister Kenny couldn't come anymore. I guess there were so many people who were coming into Sheltering Arms Hospital and Abbott Hospital in Minneapolis that she couldn't come all the way over to St. Paul. My mom felt really terrible about it. She didn't know what to do, but there really wasn't anything she could do.

A little later though, a nurse came in, and she told me, "We've got to clean you up and comb your hair. You're going for another ride." I thought, "Oh my God. What now?" Well, she said, "They're transferring you over to Minneapolis General Hospital." So they cleaned me up and brought me over there, but this time they didn't cover up my face with the rubber sheet, which was quite a relief!

When I got to Minneapolis General, they put me in this big ward with maybe 25 or 30 men. But I was the only one on that ward who had polio, at least at first. The rest of them had broken backs, broken arms, broken legs. One poor guy had fallen into a brick pile and would never get out of that bed again. We also had a city fireman on the floor with us. He had a broken leg, and they set it and put him on that ward, and he was mighty unhappy about it. He took a look at the

30 other guys in that ward and said, "How the hell are you supposed to get any sleep around here." I said, "Just close your eyes. There's nothing else you can do."

I don't remember exactly how long I was on that ward, but they used to take me twice a day to get the hot packs and exercises. Sister Kenny came to General Hospital and taught the nurses what to do. Her adopted daughter, Mary Stewart, helped with the training too. So, even though Sister Kenny didn't work with me anymore, I still got her treatment.

Eventually, they moved me to a polio ward, in other words, a ward with all polio patients. There was this one nurse on that ward, Mrs. Tupper was her name, and she was the best nurse. She knew every one of us by our first names. When she would work the night shift, Mrs. Tupper would take all the young kids out on the porch and read them stories. And if the little kids would start to cry or something, she would just pick them up and hold them, and they'd stop crying. She was the best nurse we ever had.

I remember that life was pretty regimented on that floor. Breakfast was over at 7:30 A.M., and by 8:00 A.M. you would get your hot pack, and then they would take you over to the annex where they'd do the therapy. They'd take you up to the sixth floor, and if you had an exercise bath, they'd put you in that. Sometimes you were put on a table and did your exercises there. They made me do exercises using my fingers and my toes and then my arms and legs. You'd try to make your leg work, and you'd concentrate and concentrate, and after a while you could feel it moving. It took time, of course, but I suppose every day I was improving. They didn't work on your whole body at one time. Rather, they'd focus on one specific part of your body, and when that became functional and useful again, they'd move on to another part. Since I must have spent about 11 months there at General Hospital, they had plenty of time to work on all the different parts!

I spent my birthday there and even Christmas. I remember at Christmas the V.F.W. or somebody brought in this dog, and it jumped all over the beds and everything. But the nurses didn't mind. After all, it was Christmas.

Getting back to my exercises, one day toward the end of my stay in the hospital, Bill, my physical therapist, said to me, "When we're done with your exercises today, you're going to walk around this table." I told him that I couldn't do it, and he said, "Don't think about it; just do it." Now he wasn't rough or tough or anything, but when he told you to do something, you did it. That was his job. So, when my exercises were over, I walked around the table a couple of times. Bill said, "See, you can do it." I said, "Yeah, but I was holding onto the table." Well, his response was, "I don't care if you were holding on or not. I told you to walk around the table, and you did it. You're not going back to your room in a wheelchair, you're going to walk back. I'm going to help you, but you're going to walk back." He put his arm on top of my shoulder, and I was walking down the hall. I got to this guy named Henry's room (he's the one who gets all the credit for being Sister Kenny's first patient in the U.S.), and Henry said, "Hey Bobby, you're walking." I said, "Yeah, ain't it nice. Bill's helping me." Henry looked at me and said, "Bill who?" I said, "You know, Bill, my therapist." Well, Henry kept looking at me, and finally he said, "Where is he?" And I looked around, and there was Bill, down the hall, talking to a couple of pretty, young nurses. I was walking by myself, and I didn't even know it! Well, I took three steps forward, then two steps back, and I fell flat on my butt! Henry and I were laughing so damned hard that everybody came running over, because nobody ever laughed on that ward. They all wanted to see what happened, and they were shouting, "Anybody hurt; anybody hurt?" Henry was laughing so hard he was crying, and I was just sitting on the floor laughing. But from then on, I walked.

Not too long after that, I went home. I don't remember the exact date. It was in the summer of 1941, and I walked out. I walked with a limp. They couldn't get my right foot to be completely right, so I waddled on that foot, kind of like a duck. I used a cane, just for balance, but I didn't have any braces. It took me 11 months, but when I left that damned hospital, I walked out.

After I got out of the hospital, I just stayed home for a while. I should have graduated from high school in 1941, but of course, I had spent almost that whole year in the hospital. And I didn't get to go back to school right away after I got home either. There were no handicapped students in my high school, and they told my parents that they didn't have things squared away down at the school yet. So for a while they sent a teacher out to the house a couple of times a week to give me my assignments. I don't think it was until after the first of the year that they finally said I could come back to school; they had two classes I could take. They put both of those classes in my old home room on the first floor. My dad had to take me down there every morning and then come back and pick me up about two hours later.

I must have gone there about two months or so, and then I started thinking that I better learn to do something for a living. So I went down and took this test, and they told me that I could be a draftsman or a salesman if I wanted to. Well, I didn't like the idea of being a salesman, but being a draftsman sounded all right, so I transferred to a vocational school. They were giving the same two classes I was taking at my old high school at the vocational school, and I just transferred everything over there.

I went there for almost two years. I went on Saturday mornings and only had a one week summer vacation so that I could finish the drafting course in 23 months instead of the usual 36 months.

Everyone treated me really well there. If I needed any help, all I had to do was ask for it. I remember one day the elevator didn't work, and I walked up three flights of stairs. Everybody yelled like hell, "Why didn't you say something? We would've carried you up." But the elevator got fixed, and I sure didn't want anybody to have to carry me.

Outside of school though, sometimes people would look at me like I had some kind of contagious disease. I remember one incident that happened in about 1942 or 1943, some time during the war. I had gone to the movies. I think it was at the old State Theater in downtown Minneapolis. After the movie, I was leaning up against the wall waiting for my friend to get the car, and this guy came up to me, and he was looking at me real funny. Finally, he said, "Let me see your billfold." Well, I didn't know what he was talking about, so I wasn't going to show it to him. But, he said, "I'm a Treasury Agent, and you had better show me your billfold, or you're in trouble. I want to see your draft classification. Why aren't you in the service?"

He didn't know that I had trouble walking because I was leaning up against the wall. I must've had my cane behind me, so he couldn't see it. But, believe me; I wasn't any draft dodger. Everybody in my family was in the service, all the way from my brother to every one of my cousins. I would have given my right arm to be in the military, but who knows? I could have gotten killed in the service. And if I'd gone, I probably wouldn't have met my wife, so I guess the best came out of it.

As far as other aspects of my life, I've always liked to say that polio didn't affect me that much once I had finished school. But my wife maintains that every time there was a promotion at work, somebody else always got it instead of me because of my handicap. Maybe she's right. If I'd ask why somebody else got the promotion, they'd always say, "Oh, you can't walk very good." I'd say, "Well, you don't have to walk to be a good draftsman," and their response would be, "What if you need to go out in the shop or something." Well, there were five other guys who could've gone out in the shop. I fought that for 24 years, but it's all just water over the dam now.

My first boss had been a full colonel in the Army, and he was so used to seeing men who were physically perfect that he couldn't tolerate seeing an imperfect person. But, of course, I had been hired while he was away in the war. So he couldn't figure out why they had hired me. You know, that they had hired me for my brain, not my legs, so he finally ended up firing me. But that was so long ago. That's something that I put in the past. It's a sad thing, but his son ended up getting polio. Maybe you get retribution for what you do in life.

I don't think that my disability really changed anything as far as my relationship with my wife and children. Our daughter Louisie is our third oldest. When she was in school (she must've been really little), the teacher said to her, "Your dad is Bob Gurney. He's the one who is handicapped." Well, Louisie told her, "No he's not. He's my daddy!" So I guess it didn't bother her. Even my grandkids hardly seem to notice. My oldest granddaughter always calls me "bumpa." One time our daughter took her to see the doctor, and a nurse was coming down the elevator with an empty wheelchair, and she saw that and started hollering, "Bumpa, bumpa, bumpa!" I guess she thought if there was a wheelchair, grandpa had to be in it. But we never made a big deal out of it, so our kids and our grandkids never made a big deal out of it either.

As far as the wheelchair, I guess that I started using it about 10 or 15 years ago. It was sort of a gradual thing. I started using it on and off, like when we went to Disneyland, so I wouldn't slow anyone else down. I remember that we took it with us to Canada, though not the first few times. I think the first few times when we went to Canada I just got one there from the Red Cross when I needed to use it. I used to use crutches sometimes too, but then I fell and hurt my ankle. That's when I started to rely more on the wheelchair.

I did go back to Sister Kenny Institute a number of years ago and saw a doctor there to see if there was anything that could be done about my situation. I guess that was around 1971 or 1972. At that time, I was having pain and weakness, and our family doctor said it was arthritis. I don't remember the name of the doctor I saw at Sister Kenny, but it was one of the men I knew from back when I was at General Hospital. When he examined me, he kept pointing to different muscles and saying, "This muscle is doing a job it isn't designed to do." That was the problem. The muscles that took over just couldn't do the job anymore. They were saying, "That's enough." They had done the job as long as they could, but they finally got so weak that they gave up.

The doctor didn't say I had post-polio syndrome or anything. I don't even think that they had named that yet. To this day, our family doctor won't say that's what I have. Whatever I know about post-polio syndrome, I learned through articles in the newspaper. But it's too late to worry about that now. After all, I'm going to be 70 years old in May, and I'm just thankful for the 52 years that I had after coming out of the hospital. I'm still alive! I've got four grown kids who are all doing well. I own a house, a car, and have a couple of bucks in the bank. What else do you need?

Richard Owen, M.D.

I had polio in 1940. Since I was 12 years old then, I can remember many of the details about it. Polio is an unusual disease in that there are two periods of illness as the virus enters the system. The first is associated with an infection of the nose and throat and sometimes the stomach. I had an illness that lasted for a few days, and I was even ill enough to stay home from school. I felt well the next day though, so I went back to school and carried my newspaper route. The following day, however, I was feeling ill again. I got up for breakfast and then went right back to bed. After an hour or so, I woke up and tried to get out of bed but fell to the floor because my legs would no longer move me, and I was rather limp. I was then taken to the University Hospital in Indianapolis where I was diagnosed with polio.

At that time they had some idea that it was an infectious disease, so I was given what was called "convalescent serum" which was made from the blood of people who had recovered from polio. That form of treatment was in vogue back then. It seems unlikely that it had any effect since the disease progressed to rather pronounced paralysis with no movement in either leg and no movement in my abdominal muscles. I was put in isolation, and I think I might've been told that I had poliomyelitis. However, I didn't know what poliomyelitis was. Nobody told me that I had infantile paralysis, which I would have recognized because Roosevelt was president at that time, and I knew he had suffered significant paralysis from the disease.

During my stay in the hospital, I developed appendicitis which was very difficult to diagnose because my fever had started to go down some and then I suddenly became quite ill again. The kind of signs that typically appear with appendicitis were missing because my abdominal muscles were paralyzed. As my white count went up and my stomach got distended, they finally made the diagnosis of appendicitis. It was quite an exciting trip to the operating room. I was treated like someone who had some horrible disease, and although I was coming from isolation to an operating room, there was a big crowd forming because I had this strange condition of polio complicated by appendicitis.

The two conditions are probably medically independent, but in that era I was told that 12 patients the previous year had appendicitis and polio. The polio virus is a gastrointestinal virus during part of its course, so it is conceivable that there might be some relationship between the two. But anyway, that was a side light that made my stay in the hospital exciting.

Something else that I remember very well is that I was wide awake at night and very sleepy during the day for the first couple of weeks of my hospitalization. It turns out that people with polio frequently had encephalitis, an inflammation of the brain which results in that reversal of the day/night experience. Now, years later, we're finding that some of the late effects of polio (post-polio syndrome) are probably due to the inflammation of the brain at the time of the acute illness.

In the 1940's, about 1947 or 1948, there was a man at John's Hopkins University, David Bodian, who worked with apes and corpses of people who had died from polio. He found that there had often been significant damage to the lower part of the brain, which has to do with arousal, temperature control, some degree of pain, and is also closely related to the pituitary where the connection to stress access is located. These were interesting side lights, and I don't think physicians and researchers thought about polio's effect on the brain until Dr. Bodian's studies.

It was thought that there were three types of polio: bulbar, which was toward the base of the brain; high spinal, which involved the muscles of respiration; and regular spinal, which involved weakness in the arms or the legs. It's probable that encephalitis was also a major factor in a number of people's illnesses.

Encephalitis may have also been a primary cause of death for some polio patients. The incidence of death was relatively low when the people with bulbar polio were well managed, as long as they could be kept from choking to death. That was the most common thing; the next most common thing was lack of oxygen. When we had our last epidemic at the Sister Kenny Institute in 1958 or 1959, after the development of the Salk Vaccine, we had 8 people out of 100 die, our worst statistic ever. Most of the people had a mid-brain kind of encephalitis that made it impossible to control their blood pressure and made it very difficult to phase their breathing with a respirator.

Getting back to my own illness, I was treated by the immobilization techniques that were used before Sister Kenny came to the United States and before her program was well accepted. As part of my treatment, I was kept on a frame made of canvas strapped across a metal bar.

I was then put in Toronto splints, which were leather covered splints that kept the knees bent, the feet pulled out a little bit, and the legs spread apart. It was really creative, and in some ways it was like a bad normal posture. It was almost as if the people in health care in that day and age thought normal posture should be like Leonardo da Vinci's picture of a man spread out rather than with one's legs held underneath.

I spent a total of nine months in that situation with very little therapy. The next year they did start doing therapy with me using braces and having me stand as the main form of treatment. I was also fitted with my first leg braces which weighed about 15 pounds. My present long leg brace, which I wear on my left leg, weighs only about one and a half pounds, so we've made some significant advances.

When I got out of the hospital, I was wearing one long leg brace as well as one short one, and I was using two crutches. I received some additional therapy, and I think that my mother took my therapy and rehabilitation as a very important responsibility, providing the transportation to the hospital and things like that. She gave me a lot of support, and I think she and my father were very much interested in me feeling like I was leading a normal life and that there wasn't anything I couldn't do. Though I appreciated that, it also contributed very much to a sense of denial regarding my disability that persisted for many years.

I was kept out of some things that probably facilitated my

continuing denial. For instance, I wasn't sent to a school for crippled children, and yet there was one in Indianapolis. Instead, I attended a regular school where I was the only disabled person in a student body of about 3,000. So that was quite an experience for me, and I think it was an experience for the school as well.

Back then, of course, things like architectural barriers were not of interest to anybody, not even in a school building. I had to climb a rather long flight of stairs without a railing which was pretty scary. And I had to plan my trips to the bathroom because the bathroom was in the basement as was the case in many old public schools. The stairs were metal and often times slippery from rain, so I had to be very cautious.

As far as interpersonal relationships, I had my polio at age 12, and during the year that I was out of school, all the people were maturing. The men were growing beards, and the women were growing, well, more womanly characteristics, so it was a very strange experience. It was sort of a Rip Van Winkle-type thing of being away and then coming back and finding all these people had changed.

I had also become a slow-moving person, and that was something that was really difficult for me, particularly in high school. I ended up walking alone much of the time. In a way though, that was probably all right too.

Some other important changes occurred because of my illness and subsequent disability. Before my polio, I was constantly in trouble, and I fought to and from school. I never felt that any of it was my fault. Rather, I would think that I was an innocent victim of misfortune. Also, I think I had only read about three books in my whole life up to that time, and when I compare that to my own children's reading experience where they just devoured books, it's just a fascinating thing to think that perhaps polio changed my entire life's course. I don't think I would have settled down until rather late in life, if I would have settled down at all. Before polio, I loved to fight, and I loved to play football and baseball and things like that, so there were many things that were changed because of my illness. I saw that it was impractical to fight, because I couldn't catch anybody if they ran away.

Instead of sports and fighting, I started to put my energies into my studies. I could no longer compete on the athletic field, but I could compete in the classroom. Therefore, I think polio made me into more of a scholar after my first 12 years of being very unscholarly.

It made me want to do better than other people in school because I wanted to prove myself. If I hadn't had polio, I probably wouldn't have gone to medical school, and I have no idea what else I might have done for a career.

I was headed for nothing except recreation and messing around, and that was a time when you had to make awfully good grades to get into medical school. I wasn't making good grades in elementary school, of course, and I don't think I would have done well until I was about 25 or 30 years old. Back then, late bloomers weren't nearly as well tolerated by society or family as they are now. So it would be impossible to say what sort of a career I might have had if I hadn't contracted polio. I loved to be out of doors; I loved nature. I enjoyed the kind of nature that could have led to a career in zoology or botany, and I find that still in the background of my interests, so it may well have been that a career in one of those fields would've been a natural thing for me.

Anyway, about two years after my acute illness, Elizabeth Kenny paid a visit to Indiana. That would have been in the early part of 1943 or maybe the later part of 1942. They needed some polio patients for her to work with, so she actually examined me, which was a fascinating experience. She was a large woman who wore black clothes just like in her pictures. She had a big black hat, and she wore the sort of black hose that older women wore in those days.

As she examined me, they were taking pictures right and left, and I was very fearful that I was going to appear in the newspaper wearing very little clothing. Her vision of treatment clothing was a tiny loin cloth. By good fortune, the newspaper article just said that Sister Kenny took this person (me), and got him to take a few faltering steps, which was all right. I didn't mind that because it didn't show a picture of me. After she left though, I quickly put my clothes and my brace back on and went back to high school. You can imagine how fearful a 14 or 15-year-old would be of appearing in the newspaper wearing only a loin cloth. That one incident was my only connection with Sister Kenny until 1957 when I came to Minneapolis to work at the Kenny Institute.

The staff at Indiana University had spent some time training in Minneapolis at the Sister Kenny Institute in 1942, and Kenny's visit to Indiana was related to that training. After that, the University Hospital started using the Kenny method of hot packs, stretching, and retraining muscle control, which was very different than the treatment I had received.

As I later came to realize, Sister Kenny's ideas were immensely different from the prevailing forms of treatment being used in the 1930's and 1940's. Before the Kenny method, it was thought that a muscle couldn't be retrained once it had lost its strength, and the thought was that muscle training was some unreliable fashion trend and that loss was unretrievable in the presence of disease. Sister Kenny's vision opposed this notion, believing that through blocking the message, people could actually get some recovery from at least part of the paralysis. At that time it was thought you were basically stuck where you were at about the end of one year, yet recovery actually takes place over a couple of years.

Sister Kenny also had a great dislike for bracing, and she thought that there were certain kinds of crutches you could use that would encourage you to walk better. She used techniques that challenged you to use the muscle that you had. For instance, her parallel bars were two-by-fours, rather than the usual round gadgets you could grab a hold of. It hadn't occurred to me until I got into medicine the impact the difference had because if you're walking along with bars to hold on to and grasp, you can actually pull yourself forward on the bars and propel yourself along. If you use two-by-fours, however, you have to bear weight through your legs and through your hands.

Getting back to my own situation, by 1945 when I graduated from high school, I was walking with a cane, and I had gotten rid of my long leg brace. A couple of years later, I think it was in 1947, I had surgery on my foot to stabilize my left ankle. That made it possible for me to walk a little bit better than I had been, and I walked with a cane but without bracing for an extended period of time.

When I went to college, I had to do a lot of planning in advance for my walking because I was at Indiana University, which is a huge campus with a lot of ups and downs and hills and lovely wooded trails between buildings. Of course, most of the buildings did not have accessible entry points at that time, so I learned a lot about planning ahead and being late to class. I also found out that at a big university, there's very little attention paid to individual students, which was quite a contrast to my high school where I was the only disabled person in a very large school, and where all of my teachers knew about my disability. At Indiana University, I couldn't charm my professors or make them feel any sympathy for me. Therefore, I had to suddenly start working.

Actually, the whole experience of being a disabled adolescent is weird. There's a lot more dependence on fantasy and scenario writing. It's interesting, but I think in some ways my experiences as a disabled adolescent made me a more effective person in medical management areas because I tend to be much more a person who visualizes and has some degree of intuition. I also plan ahead just like I had to plan ahead for going to the bathroom in grade school. I still have to plan a lot of my activities.

When I got into medical school, I was still walking without any bracing, but I had to spend a lot of time standing and a lot of time walking. I went to medical school in Washington D.C., and there were a lot of places I wanted to go and things I wanted to see. So, by the end of my freshman year, I started to wear a brace again because it was a lot more comfortable for me. Elizabeth Kenny would've thought it was a bad idea, but when you balance out function as opposed to what she thought was normal gait, I had to go for function.

After I finished my medical training in 1957, I accepted a position at the Sister Kenny Institute in Minneapolis. I had no intention of coming to the Kenny Institute to work. Rather, I was heading west, or so I thought. But we bumped into some very nice people at Sister Kenny, and I decided to take a position here. That decision turned out well for me. I worked at the Kenny Institute until I retired in 1993.

It's interesting that I ended up working here because I made no particular connection in my mind between working at Sister Kenny and my polio or even the fact that I had met Sister Kenny. At that point in my life, I was still in a stage where I was pretty much denying that I had anything wrong, and that was really the way I felt until I was about 45 years old.

I find my denial an interesting thing now because I've looked at the sociology of it. For many years, I didn't think there was much wrong with me. My vision of myself was of a person who was just maybe one step behind everybody else physically, but equal in every other way. However, other people didn't see me in that same way. For instance, I went to my 35th reunion of my medical school class. I hadn't been back for 35 years because it hadn't really interested me, but it was really fascinating when we all got up to tell our stories of something that was interesting to us when we were in medical school. To my surprise, two or three people talked about me and my example of extraordinary bravery and courage.

That struck me as so odd that when I got up to say my piece, I needed to respond to some of those comments. I said that when I was in medical school, my denial mechanisms were so strong that courage was probably the last word I would have used to describe myself as far as dealing with my physical handicap. Rather, I was very competitive, and I was just trying to keep up with my medical school classmates. I think that's why I decided to take a surgical internship. I wanted to prove once more that I could do it. It was part of my drive to prove that there wasn't anything wrong with me, and then years later I discovered that people were thinking I was courageous to do it. It was a dumb thing to do, and I learned that lesson after about three or four months, but I also found that I liked some of the aspects of surgery in that I could see a problem and work toward the solution.

I've found that in rehabilitation there are many similarities to surgery. You don't have the emergency. You're not going to have an artery rupture that you'd better be clamping or sewing, but in rehabilitation, I can see a problem, like with strength or range of motion, and I can take a look at anatomy or watch a walk and do an analysis of something that requires my thinking and gives me a chance to respond and correct the problem. That's very different than trying to prescribe the right medication for the right disease and have the person respond correctly to that medication.

At any rate, when I got into rehabilitation, I experienced another twist of finding that people thought I understood them because I was also disabled. Yet, I wasn't really in touch with them, and I wasn't really responding to them because I understood myself and my disability. Rather, I understood what the image of myself was doing to our relationship. So it was a weird twist that made it possible for me to enjoy a position of acceptance quickly, and yet I wasn't really empathizing with them as another person with a disability. Still, it's been a connection for me to people with all sorts of disabling conditions because there's a barrier broken when the physician or the counselor or whoever, has a disability. It is a lot less of a threat to a person.

There've been some good studies on that, where counselors who had disabilities were studied as opposed to counselors who weren't disabled. Often, the barriers to counseling were broken down faster because there's less fear of a physical threat, or maybe it's just a sense that somebody understands a painful experience or vulnerability. So, the person you're counseling sees it as an empathetic situation much more quickly and then because of that, has a sense of security.

I remember one time when a real strange man with a spinal cord injury came to see me. He got to talking to me, and he was looking at my head, right at the top of my forehead, which gave me an uncomfortable feeling. Finally, he said, "I can see you have the mark of sorrow on your forehead." At first I thought he said, the mark of "Zoro!" But he was saying that he thought I had the mark of sorrow on my forehead. And it was such an odd thing, because I don't have a sorrowful feeling for myself. I think he was responding to me that way because I limped into the room or used a brace, so we had sort of a connection.

I also think when I stand up to make a speech on the subject of disability, there's a feeling that I speak with some authority just because I've been there too. I know what a weak muscle feels like, and I know what a muscle that needs stretching feels like. So it gives me an advantage in some circumstances.

My own post-polio problems have given me a connection to other post-polio patients with whom I've worked. They know that I'm experiencing some of the same things, and so they're more likely to listen to me and accept my recommendations.

Actually, my post-polio syndrome started at about the time it should have, 30 years after my polio in 1970, but it wasn't a recognized phenomenon then. I thought it was maybe just that I was de-conditioned or that I was so busy with my career that I really wasn't paying attention to a decay of function. And the decay of function that I was experiencing was additional weakness. About that same time, and maybe even preceding it, I started to modify the things I did in my life as I had increasing responsibilities with family and increasing responsibilities in medicine; so I stopped doing some of the physical things that I had done a lot of before. I less often went camping, less often went to Canada, things like that.

I'm not sure if I cut back on some things unintentionally in advance, but maybe subtly because of post-polio, or maybe it led to post-polio by cutting down on physical activities. I think there's probably a little bit of both in post-polio syndrome. Some people give up functions that they wish they had back, and we know that part of the problem is that a polio muscle that's weak needs to be trained up to a very high functional level. That's in contrast to a person without polio who might have a 75% reserve in the muscle, and might at their hardest use about 75% of their musculature at a given time in an activity. The people with polio are often times using about 90 to 100% of their capacity in their daily activities, so if you undertrain for a bit, you develop weakness from that undertraining. That's very significant, and I think that happens to a lot of people who had polio. I think that's probably at least a part of what happened with me.

I've not had problems with fatigue, but that might be denial. And I haven't had pain, but I don't think that I know much about pain personally, because more often than not when I have pain, it's because of something I've done to myself when I'm out having fun. I don't really suffer from that. For instance, when I played wheelchair basketball, my arms would be stiff and sore in the morning, but it's never been really painful.

I had a friend at Ohio State who said that the football players, if they lost a game, would all come in and have therapy and massage. If they won the game, they wouldn't see them. So, winners celebrate, and losers have pain. Along the same line, I think that if you're imposing the pain on yourself, you find it more acceptable than if it's imposed by some other thing or destiny. I'm sure that if I had rheumatoid arthritis, I'd be terribly upset at the fact that this was done to me by some disease.

I think the biggest problem I currently have as a result of polio and my post-polio problems is reduced accessibility to places that I would like to visit. For instance, I don't see myself going to Rome, or going to Moscow, or going to some of the old countries and old spots in Europe because of accessibility.

We were in England recently, and I used my wheelchair there, and it was a fascinating experience because so few people seemed to be out in wheelchairs. Yet parts of the old sections of London were actually shaped for carts to go up and down on the sidewalks. So there were a lot of ramps in the old parts of England. But I think lack of accessibility is the thing that I mind the most.

The impact of polio on my life hasn't been totally negative. I've already mentioned some of the positive effects on my education, career, and connections to others with disabilities. As far as other things, I think polio has given me a chance to be in wheelchair athletics, particularly wheelchair basketball. Because of that, I've had a great variety of people as friends that as a doctor I wouldn't necessarily have met. So, I have a life that's in that arena, and I have a life at home, and a life as a disabled person, and a life as an able-bodied person in medicine. That's made things very interesting for me.

Something else that's interesting, to me at least, is the impact that my disability has had on my children. I think my disability has given them a different experience too. My daughter, for example, married one of the spinal-cord-injured fellows on my wheelchair basketball team, and they have been terribly happy. She's very sensitive to accessibility and mobility needs, and they have a very loving relationship. I think that her connection with a sense that I, as her father, and my wife, as her mother, worked through a relationship that had the complications of a physical disability helped with that.

My oldest son is in psychiatry. He went to medical school, and his experience was that he had shared some of my friendships with disabled people. He also saw me as a person in that realm of medicine. So I think maybe that helped him in his career.

My youngest son was the ball boy on our wheelchair basketball team. The first few times we went on the road we would sleep in a motel room, and the person in the room with us would be a spinal-cord-injured person. That made his life a very fascinating experience, and resulted in him becoming very accepting of a variety of people to the extent that he would talk about his teachers at school, and we'd have no idea what their race was or if they had any disabilities. Then we'd go to PTA and find, for example, that he had a very charming black woman as a teacher who wore African dresses. So he was very accepting of a diversity of people.

My experiences as a disabled person have sometimes been amusing too because I've had the pleasure of experiencing the sociology of a disability from both worlds. When I go around a lake, people will say things like, "Oh, it's nice that you're able to be out," but sometimes they will feel uncomfortable and look away, and I get a sense that I know what passes through their minds. Seeing me suggests a potential frailty in all of us that a lot of people don't want to admit. I've seen that in some of my friends as they've grown older. Perhaps they've been athletes or runners, and they've told me that they have knee problems or hip problems or back problems, and they have to give up running or some other activity that has been an important part of their life. And they feel such a sense of despair. Whereas I've already taken care of that despair, so it puts me in an interesting position.

Ray K. Gullickson

I was raised on a farm near the small town of Cushing in western Wisconsin. Late in the summer of 1946, when I was 16 years old, my older brother and I were left in charge of the farm while our parents went on a vacation. They had no definite itinerary, but they planned to visit some relatives, and they would be gone for a month or six weeks. They left money for our expenses and said they would call us from time to time.

One of the assignments we were given before my father left was to build a temporary, electric fence around one of the grain fields. We had already harvested the crop from that field, and we were fencing it off to add some additional pasture land where we could graze cattle. The system we were using involved driving lightweight, wooden posts into the ground, putting insulators on them, and then stringing a single, barbed wire from insulator to insulator all around the field. The wire was charged with electricity, and if the animals touched the wire they would get a shock. They learned very quickly to stay within the fenced area, and after a day or two with the charger running, we didn't even have to turn it on anymore.

My brother was 10 years older than I was, and he liked to be the boss and assign the tasks. He decided that my job was to pound in the posts, and he would string the wire. I knew he was taking advantage of me, but I didn't mind. I was confident I could keep ahead of him, and I took a great deal of pride in doing my share of the work. On that day, I pounded in more than 140 fence posts.

Because it was rather dry that August and our clay soil was very hard, I had to use a heavy sledge hammer with a three-foot wooden handle and a 16 pound head. We started right after breakfast, and it made for a long and grueling day, but by about six that evening, we had finished the fence.

Following that work, my brother asked me to help him install the drive wheel on one of the farm machines. The wheel weighed close to 150 pounds, and the machine weighed about a ton. We fashioned a lever and fulcrum to lift one side of the machine. Because my brother was 20 pounds heavier than I was, he served as the weight on one end of a plank, while I slid the wheel onto the axle. That was the last thing I remember doing that day because right after lifting the wheel, I collapsed.

My brother took me to the Grantsburg Hospital where my sister worked as a practical nurse. If I had remained there, the doctor would have subjected me to his plan of treatment, which involved using Swedish massage. Fortunately, my sister had worked at Shriner's Hospital in Portland, Oregon, and she had seen a lot of polio patients there. She recognized my symptoms and decided that Grantsburg Hospital wasn't the place for me. When the doctor went home for dinner, my sister telephoned my brother and said, "We have to get Ray out of here, right away." In defiance of the doctor's plan, and without any real authority, she discharged me on her own volition. I am eternally grateful that she had the courage to do this, or I might have been crippled all my life.

My brother laid me on the back seat of his car and took me to Minneapolis General Hospital where they did a spinal tap and confirmed the diagnosis. The next morning, I was admitted to Station K, which was the Sister Kenny ward. I met my roommate, Warren S. I was very weak and tired, so I didn't have much of a conversation with him, but I learned that he was a press operator for the Minneapolis Star newspaper.

A few minutes later, I was lying very still when someone came into the room and pulled the bedsheet up over my face. I thought nothing of it until later that day, when Warren asked me again what my name was. Then, saying nothing, he handed me his copy of the afternoon paper and pointed to a report of polio-fatalities on the front page. I found my name listed among the dead.

Meanwhile, my sister had managed to contact my parents, somewhere in New England, and my mother was flying home. My cousin Bill was listening to the local news on the car radio as he drove to the airport to meet her. When he heard my name and a report that I had died from polio, he was alarmed but decided not to become the bearer of bad news. He turned off the radio and didn't say anything to my mother. She came to the hospital, but Station K was isolated for contagion, so visitors were not allowed inside.

Fortunately, my mother was spared the news of my "death." By the time she arrived, the charge nurse had discovered her error. It turned out that the nurse had read my name on the clip-board at the foot of my bed while I was covered, like a corpse, under the sheet. Thinking that I was dead, she reported my death to the newspaper and WCCO Radio.

I only stayed at General Hospital for a couple of days. Then I was transferred to the Fort Snelling Army Post where Sister Kenny patients were being cared for in an old barracks building. It was a 40 bed ward, and we were treated by Army doctors with the help of a lot of volunteers and a small nursing staff. Everyone was exhausted from working too hard, but I thought that the quality of care that we received there was very good.

The next day, I met Sister Kenny, and I saw her several times a week when she came for morning "rounds" with the doctors and a Kenny therapist. The treatment at Fort Snelling was the typical Sister Kenny approach where the patient is wrapped in hot packs. The packs were made of heavy woolen cloth, and there was a layer of rubber sheeting on the outside to keep them in place. They were heated in a boiler and spun-dried to remove most of the water, but they were still very hot, about 140 degrees, when they were placed on our bare skin. One of the volunteer packers told us that the temperature of the packs shouldn't exceed 150 degrees, or we would be scalded. The treatment continued, all day and all night, 24 hours a day, and as soon as we started to cool off, they'd put on another set of packs.

Several times a week, I was also taken to a small treatment room where I would receive therapy. Occasionally, Sister Kenny would participate in the therapy session, but most of the time someone else would help me exercise my arms and legs and other affected parts of my body. I don't know how long those therapy sessions lasted, but I remember I was always very tired when they were over, and I wanted to go back to my bed.

The patients were also responsible for part of the therapy. For example, there was a footboard on everyone's bed, and we were told to keep our feet up against that board. They told me only once, and I was expected to remember and do it even if I didn't understand why it was important. It was a very uncomfortable posture.

A few days after I got to Fort Snelling, I heard Sister Kenny telling a new patient to use the footboard. She was saying exactly the same things I had been told, so I thought to myself, "Well, if this is a rule, and it's important enough to be given in the same way to every patient, then I'd better be doing it." I asked her what would happen if I didn't keep my feet against the board. She replied that I might develop "drop foot." That meant the tight muscles in my legs would change the angle of my foot, causing it to drop, and my toes would drag when I tried to walk. From then on, I made sure I was doing everything Sister Kenny and the therapist told me to do. If they said something was important, I tried to learn why, and then I did it.

I have some really vivid memories of Sister Kenny. She was a very tall and elegant woman, and she inspired confidence just by her manner and by the way she carried herself. She had a delightful accent which made her a fascinating person to listen to. If I close my eyes, I can still visualize her standing next to my bed wearing a long, black dress and a big hat with a beautiful ostrich feather. I once heard her tell someone that the plume in her hat was selected and dyed just for her, to match the color of her hat. She didn't wear jewelry, and she didn't wear any makeup. I remember her face as being strong and angular, and her eyes were very intense. When she looked you in the eye, that intensity demanded all of your attention, and when she spoke, people listened to her.

She made rounds with the Army doctors, and she took a personal interest in every patient. I remember that one of those doctors was very outspoken. He would make his observations about the patient's condition and begin to tell the therapist how he thought things should be done. At first Sister Kenny would listen, but if she didn't agree, she would raise her voice and talk louder than the doctor. She'd say what she had to say, and when she was finished, she'd just walk away. Everyone knew that she was in charge, and we received whatever treatment she recommended. I've never known anyone as assertive as she was.

Probably because I had used my right arm and leg so extensively on the day that I came down with polio, my paralysis was all on my right side. When my therapy began, Sister Kenny explained to me exactly what they were going to do and how they were going to accomplish it. She took my right hand in hers and pointed to a muscle in my wrist. As she tapped the muscle with her finger tip, she told me that muscle was the one we were going to start with, and when that muscle started to work, we'd do another and another until we got them all working. She showed me how to touch my thumb with my finger tips, and she told me to repeat the exercise until I was too tired to continue. Of course, I couldn't do it at first, but finally I got to the point where I was able to do it quickly and steadily for a minute or longer, and that was very encouraging.

While I continued to work on strengthening my right hand and wrist, I was getting other therapy as well. I was learning to lift my knee off the bed, pull my leg back, and then put it down again. Though every little bit of progress was as exciting as hitting a homerun, the main turning point for me occurred during a therapy session where they started to stretch my muscles.

On that day, I went to therapy with one of the doctors, Sister Kenny, a therapist, and maybe a couple of attendants. On the way down there, they told me that they were going to stretch me. I didn't know what to expect, but I was encouraged because my right leg was about two and one-half inches shorter than the left, and my back muscles were so tight that it was like having a "charley horse" cramp that persisted, day and night, without any relief.

On the way to treatment, Sister Kenny said, "Most people find the stretching very painful," but then she explained how to manage the pain. She said, "Pain is just a signal from your body that something is wrong. Once you recognize why it is happening, you don't need to feel the pain anymore." That sounded really sensible to me, so I thought, "Hey, if it means I'm making progress, I don't need to feel the pain." And that's really how I felt about it. I've been able to manage persistent pain ever since that day.

When we got to the treatment room, they put me, face down, near one end of the treatment table. My upper body was resting on the pad, and my legs were both dangling over the end. One attendant, who was a huge guy of about six foot-four inches tall, stood on one side of the table, leaned over, grabbed the other edge and held down the upper part of my body with his elbows. Another attendant got on the other side, reached across, and held my lower trunk firmly against the table. The Kenny therapist sat on the floor under the table and grasped my right leg, which was dangling over the edge with the healthy one.

Sister Kenny stood by my head and told me they would "begin the treatment" by pulling my right leg under the table. I guess they usually stretched the patient a little at a time, and they may have been expecting me to beg them to stop, but I didn't protest. So, in my case, they never let up, and there was no relief until minutes later, when they finished the treatment. Then they moved me up on the table, and Sister Kenny compared the length of my two legs. She said, "We *have it*; they're within a quarter of an inch!"

The therapist said he was surprised that I didn't make any fuss about the pain, but pain was not my predominant feeling. Admittedly, it had been an excruciating experience, but in another sense, the treatment was so exciting that I hardly felt it because it represented a victory over some of the muscle cramping I was experiencing.

I was feeling really good about the way that session had gone, and I remember that Sister Kenny also seemed very pleased. The doctor didn't say anything, but I assumed that he was also gratified with the results. Before the treatment, my back had been so badly arched that I think you could have easily rolled a baseball under me while I was lying "flat." After that one treatment, my back was straight, and my right leg had stretched back to within a quarter of an inch of the length of my left leg, which was not affected by my polio.

Later that evening, I wanted to use a telephone to call some of my relatives who lived in St. Paul. I didn't have any money to make a long distance call, so I wasn't going to call my parents, but I was pretty excited about the stretching and the rest of my progress, and I wanted to tell somebody what had happened. One of the attendants put me in a wheelchair so I could use a phone in the office of the Army doctor who had watched my treatment that day. It wasn't unusual to use the doctor's phone because there were no public phones in that barracks.

As I was getting ready to make my call, I reached for the handle of a file cabinet so that I could turn my wheelchair around. As it happened, the drawer popped open, and I saw my name on a medical file. I knew I'd be snooping, but I just couldn't resist this opportunity to look for some good news, perhaps even that I'd be able to go home pretty soon. I pulled out my chart and read it, but I couldn't believe what I saw. The doctor had written that I would not be able to walk for at least a year and that I would always need to wear some sort of a leg brace or, as he called it, an "appliance." It had never occurred to me that I wouldn't be able to walk again or that I'd need a brace, and I remember sitting there, shaking my head in utter disbelief and thinking, "Absolutely not! I will not wear a brace." With that kind of news, I was feeling so discouraged that I didn't want to talk with anyone. There was no longer any reason to call, so I got help to return to my bed.

Late that evening, after they had turned off most of the lights in the barracks, I grabbed the edge of my bed with my left hand and lowered myself onto the floor to see if I could stand up. I was very weak, and I wondered if this was such a good idea. Standing for the first time after many weeks gave me quite a sensation. It was like my feet were asleep, and I was being pricked by hundreds of tiny needles. I broke out in a cold sweat, and I started to shake. I knew I was in danger of falling, and it would take all the strength that I had left, but I was determined to climb back into bed. I remember lying there, breathless as if I'd just won a race. Of course, I hadn't even left the *starting line*, but standing on my own two feet again was such an exciting thing. I knew right then that the doctor was wrong. I was going be able to walk again, and I knew I wasn't going to need a brace.

I didn't tell anyone what I had done, but I repeated the routine every night for more than a week. Each time I tried to stand a little longer, and I could feel myself getting stronger. Within 10 days or so, I was able to take a step. A few days after that, I was able to walk completely around the end of my bed, and I still had enough strength left to climb back in. However, I still didn't tell anybody what I was doing.

Shortly after that, on a Saturday some time in November, I was trying to make a phone call to Carol, who was my girlfriend then and is now my wife, and somehow, the phone lines got crossed. I think my parents may have been calling Carol's parents, and just for a moment, I overheard my mother say that they were thinking of coming to see me. Then I got cut off, and I didn't hear the rest of the conversation. I had not seen any of my loved ones for several months because we were in isolation, but the next day, on Sunday afternoon, I was sitting in a wheelchair near the sun porch when I saw Carol coming across the parade ground near the barracks.

I forgot I was in a wheelchair, stood up, and walked over to the sun porch to meet her. It was the first time anyone had seen me walk, and I'm not sure who was the most excited: Carol, Sister Kenny, or me! I made it as far as the doorway, but then I collapsed, making a lot of racket when I struck the floor.

The doctor and the nurses seemed totally exasperated, and one of them said, "Now look what you've gone and done!" Maybe they expected me to have broken bones, but they sure weren't very careful when they picked me up and dropped me into the wheelchair. I had lost about 70 pounds, and I was just skin and bones then, so when I fell into the chair, it hurt almost as much as when I had hit the floor.

I remember that everybody was talking at once, but Sister Kenny didn't say anything. She just reached over and put her hand on my shoulder, and I could tell that she was delighted by what I had done. She knew I was eager to visit with Carol, so I didn't talk to her until the next day when she made rounds. It was then that I told her how I had learned to walk. Her reaction was one of genuine satisfaction, not only for my sake, but for the inspiration she thought I could be to others.

A few days later, Sister Kenny asked me if I would be willing to go over to the station hospital and talk to CJ, another patient who came from my hometown. She told me that in spite of having only a mild paralysis, he was not cooperating with his treatment and had just been lying in bed, feeling sorry for himself ever since he was admitted. I could tell that she had very little patience left for CJ, and it was obvious that she'd rather work with people who were willing to try and get well.

I didn't know this fellow very well, but I did go and talk to him. I explained how I felt challenged by the bad news in my chart and had decided to prove it wrong. I even stood up and walked for him, but he wasn't the least bit impressed with what I had done. That surprised me, and because I believed my recovery was closely influenced by my attitude, it was discouraging to see a young person who really didn't seem willing to help himself.

I don't know any details, but I believe part of the problem was that he would go home on weekends, and everyone would buy him drinks. Because of that, he had gained a lot of weight. I could understand why Sister Kenny might feel she was wasting her time with him. CJ left the hospital a few days after I visited him. He was never able to walk on his own and ended up needing to use Kenny sticks for the rest of his life. I heard that he died recently.

Sister Kenny believed alcohol was damaging to the nervous system, and it would impair the healing a polio patient needs in order to get well. I recall one time when a couple of patients in our barracks asked some of their Army friends to smuggle in some whiskey for them. The next morning Sister Kenny could smell it on their breath, and I heard her tell them, rather loudly, that she didn't tolerate any drinking in the hospital. She said she was willing to help them, but if they wanted to drink more than they wanted to get well, then she just didn't have any more time for them. The next day they were gone!

I think that showed the single-mindedness of purpose that Kenny had. She believed that patients should be in her facility for only one reason, to get well. She wouldn't approve of anything that interfered with that objective.

Getting back to my own situation, not very long after I started walking, probably still some time in late November, I went home. There was some confusion about my release from the hospital, and I'm not exactly sure what happened. Maybe I was supposed to be released just for the Thanksgiving holiday or a weekend visit, but I misunderstood and told my parents they could come and get me. When they came, I remember overhearing somebody on the staff trying to explain that I wasn't supposed to be permanently released, but my parents said, "Well, we came all this distance, and if he wants to go home, then we're going to take him." Of course, I did want to go home, and so I left that day. Later, I was ashamed when I learned that my chart showed I was discharged "under protest."

I did go back to the Kenny Institute a couple of times for follow-up visits, but other than that, I had no more therapy or treatment until recently when I experienced the onset of the post-polio syndrome. I had deliberately decided that I was not going to wear a brace or use a cane, and I stuck to that decision until the past 10 months. I have always kept a cane in the car, however. That way if I ever got stuck someplace where I had to do a lot of walking, I'd have one if I needed it.

I also remember that I was told I shouldn't return to school that year, but I went back a few days before the Christmas holidays. I was by no means fully recovered, and sometimes I would get so tired that I'd walk along the side of the hallway and use the wall to help support me.

We lived out in the country, so of course, I rode a school bus. The first time the bus came to pick me up, the driver brought the bus into the farm yard. Having him do that made me feel very "crippled," so every day after that, I walked the three-fourths of a mile to the bus stop. I was one of the first students to get on the bus at about 7:15 A.M., and the bus had to travel 50 or 60 miles before nine o'clock when we got to school. It was after four when I got on the bus at the end of the day, and I don't think I got home until about six. So it was a very long day. Still, I stuck it out and graduated from high school with the rest of my class in 1947. By that time, I was a lot stronger and hardly limped at all.

After high school, I enrolled at Gustavus Adolphus College where I majored in fine arts and social work. I graduated in 1951; Carol and I got married, and we've been together almost 44 years. We have three grown children and two grandchildren.

So polio didn't prevent me from going to college, getting a job, or having a normal family life, but it did keep me out of the service during the Korean conflict. I was a social worker for about five years, but I found working with people who were *willing* to be dependent very frustrating, so I quit and went into the insurance business. I was a successful agent, manager, and home-office executive until a few years ago when I started my own publishing company.

For well over 40 years, I lived a very "normal" life. My disability was only sometimes an inconvenience and did not prevent me from doing the things I needed or wanted to do. However, over this last year or so, I've started to have some new polio-related problems. They began when I was working on a book that required 200 hours of writing with a very strict deadline. I started in mid-October and finished early in December. In doing that project, I sometimes worked as long as 14 hours a day, and I'd get so caught up in my work that I would forget to eat. When I finished that project, I was totally exhausted and depressed. Worse yet, I was also experiencing a lot of pain, and I had trouble keeping my eyes in focus.

I went to my family doctor and told him how awful I was feeling. He did a bunch of blood tests and said I was in excellent health except that I had a chemical deficiency that was causing my depression. He prescribed a medication called Paxil, and within about two weeks, I was feeling a lot better. The Paxil restored my healthy mental outlook, but it didn't stop the pain, and when I drove my car, I had to keep one eye closed to prevent double vision.

I continued to have muscle cramps in my chest that were so severe, my ribs would actually come out of alignment. Also, when I became tired, my voice would give out, and my handwriting started to show some significant changes. My doctor suggested that I see a neurologist. When the neurologist finished a few tests, he confirmed that I was in excellent health, except for the fact that I had post-polio syndrome. I thought, "NO! This guy is all wrong, just like the doctor at Fort Snelling."

The neurologist sent me back to my primary care physician so that I could get a referral to be evaluated at Sister Kenny Institute. I knew very little about how post-polio syndrome progresses, so I went to a university medical library and looked it up. I learned that as many as 80% of paralytic polio patients have a recurrence of their symptoms between the ages of 45 and 55. Well, I thought that proved me right. I was already past age 60, and I had no serious signs of paralysis, so I chose to believe I was one of the 20% of polio survivors who wasn't going to get it.

When I went over to Kenny Institute, they did a lot of testing and confirmed that I do have post-polio syndrome. They would not venture any guess as to how it may affect me, but they told me it would be harmful to try to fight it, because that could damage my other muscles that have carried 70% of my weight for so many years. "In effect," they said, "the problem is that your right side had polio, and it has taken it easy for 50 years, but remember, your left side did all the work, and now it's like it would be normally at about age 95." Since then, I've had to admit that positive thinking isn't going to do the job this time.

I've taken some unexpected falls recently, and I have difficulty using drawing instruments to illustrate my books, but a new eyeglass prescription (with prisms) has reinforced my eye muscles, and I can again drive safely with both eyes open. Other signs of weakness have developed, and the painful cramping has continued. When I heard that a medication named Elavil was being used by post-polio patients, I asked the doctor to prescribe it. Elavil has helped a great deal in controlling my pain and other symptoms, including sleeplessness.

It was hard for me to accept the fact that I have to live with this condition, but I feel pretty well when I remember to rest for an hour after every two hours of work. I've decided that my post-polio symptoms *came late,* and they are *progressing slowly,* so I believe I still have a lot of great years left. *I intend to make the most of them!*

Chapter 3

Of Iron Lungs and Wheelchairs

For those old enough to remember the polio epidemics of the 1940's and 1950's, a number of images probably come to mind including March of Dimes posters, crowded hospital wards, and children wearing leg braces or walking with crutches. For many though, perhaps the most terrifying memory from that era is the iron lung. Developed in the late 1920's, it consisted of a large metal tank equipped with a pump to assist respiration by changing the pressure within the tank. When polio patients were unable to breathe on their own, they were placed inside the iron lung until they were able to regain the capacity for unassisted respiration. Some never did, and therefore, never got out.

Only two of those we interviewed recalled being placed in iron lungs. David Kangas spent just a few days in one before regaining the capacity for unassisted breathing. Marilynne Rogers, on the other hand, still requires the help of her 1950's vintage iron lung (or "respirator" as she calls it) on a daily basis. She sleeps in it, and for the most part, has done so since 1949 when she developed polio.

Marilynne and David also have something else in common. They have both needed the assistance of a wheelchair since they suffered their acute illness. Therefore, their stories give us a first-hand account not only of the iron lung, but also of what it was like to be out and about in a wheelchair long before there was any concern for handicapped accessibility. David's description of his years at the University of Minnesota presents a compelling argument for

handicapped parking and accessibility, and the fact that he has had a
good life and successful career in spite of the extent of his disability
is a study in determination and making the best of a difficult
situation.

Marilynne Rogers

I had polio in late August of 1949 when I was nine years old. I
remember that I had a terrible headache on the day I was diagnosed.
My mother called my cousin, who was a nurse, and asked her to
come over and take a look at me. They were both worried about the
possibility of polio because there was quite an epidemic that year. My
cousin came into my room where I was lying down and tried to touch
my chin to my chest and to get me to touch my head to my knees. It
was extremely painful for me. I think I went, "Aghh!" I was very
athletic then, so they were pretty sure that something was wrong.

A pediatrician was called, and he was an older doctor. He thought
I needed a spinal tap but didn't want to do it himself because of his
age. So he sent one of his young colleagues to meet us at Abbot
Hospital in Minneapolis where they did the spinal tap.   I can
remember having that done because they said it might hurt, so I was
a bit apprehensive. They had me crawl up onto a table on my
stomach, and they must've injected me with novocaine because at
first I really didn't feel it. Then the doctor said there'd be a lot of
pressure. I remember I had to lean a little to get the needle in, but I
don't remember it hurting. Later in the hospital, all the other kids
said it really hurt.

I remember the doctors talked to my parents and said I should
probably be admitted to the hospital because my cell counts weren't
good. I'm not sure what that meant about my later disability. I don't
even know if they could tell the different kinds of polio at that time.
I don't think so. Anyway, they took me to what was then called
Minneapolis General Hospital where they had a polio ward.

My parents thought I should have slippers because I didn't want to
wear shoes, so we stopped to get the slippers on our way to General
Hospital. I remember going upstairs, and I can vaguely remember the
elevator trip. Then I remember going down this big hall. It must have
been really crowded there because they took me to a room at first,
but then they took me out to a hallway. Eventually, I was put into a
room again. I think my room was on a porch. It had windows on
three sides, and it was pretty wide. I believe there were three beds

against the widest wall. The two shorter sides were just huge windows. A doctor came in and did some muscle tests, and I also remember I danced with somebody there. I was stronger than he was and had more muscle power, especially in my legs. That was the last time I ever danced.

I can vividly recall the other patients on that ward because they were wearing these awful hospital gowns which were all open in the back. I believe they also had on pajama bottoms. I can remember seeing the bandages across their backs where they obviously had the spinal tap. Although I didn't know it, I probably had a bandage on my back too.

My bed was a little bit to the right of the door, so I could look out at that long hall, and I have a really vivid memory of that first night at the hospital because I had to go to the bathroom, and I was getting weaker. I crawled out of bed, and I didn't know I was supposed to call for a nurse. It seemed to take me hours to crawl down to the other end of the hall where the bathroom was. There was a nurse's desk out in the hall, and they finally noticed me and took me back to my bed. They made me use a bed pan. I thought that was highly insulting. I wanted to go to the bathroom, but instead I got a bed pan!

The morning of the third day I was hospitalized, which was the first or second of September, I had cereal, juice, and chocolate milk for breakfast. I remember trying to pick up the chocolate milk, and it fell right through my hand. I felt so bad because I couldn't move anymore. The nurses all rushed in and cleaned up the mess. I remember I wanted the chocolate milk, but I didn't get it. Instead, they brought me a straw, and I drank some juice. After that, some doctors came into my room and had me count backwards, 10-9-8-7-6, for as long as I remember. I was lying down at that time because I was having trouble sitting up.

After a while, they came in and told me they were going to put me in a machine that would make me feel better. I would be more comfortable. I don't think they called it an iron lung or even a respirator when they were telling me about it. But I remember they wheeled me into this small room, and there was this big machine. I think because my cousin was a nurse and had been trained at the University, I wasn't really afraid of medical personnel. I rather trusted them when they told me I would feel better. I remember they opened the respirator; it seemed really huge, and they laid me on the tray with a mattress on it, and then they slid me through the hole at the front of the big roller part. Then they closed up the collar and told me to really relax. They told me I'd feel much better, and I did. I could breathe more easily.

After that, I think I pretty much lost everything. I don't really remember the sequence of events for the period that followed, so I probably was not too coherent for a while. I do remember being left on the respirator, but I have no idea for how long. According to my hospital chart, I was in and out of the respirator after the first few weeks. I know I was out of the respirator for several periods of up to five weeks. I assumed that I wouldn't need it anymore, but it didn't turn out that way. I've needed it all my life. I still sleep in it. To me, the time I spend in the respirator is the time to sleep.

At any rate, I guess that I was at General Hospital through the end of February. Then they moved me to Elizabeth Kenny Institute. That was because they got some kind of epidemic at Minneapolis General. They had to move 80 of us respirator patients out to various other hospitals. I was told at that time that the Elizabeth Kenny Institute didn't accept respirator patients, but there was kind of a rumor that they told Sister Kenny she had to accept us if the National Foundation was going to continue contributing to the Institute.

I remember going there in an ambulance because by then I could be out of the respirator for four or five hours at a time as long as I didn't have congestion. I remember my mother was with me. They took me out of the ambulance, and when we got to the door, they said parents weren't allowed. Now, at Minneapolis General Hospital, my parents could be there anytime, 24 hours a day, even on weekends. But at the Kenny Institute, I think they could be there only for two hours every Sunday, which was pretty devastating for a child.

Of course, I got the Sister Kenny treatment at the Kenny Institute. Actually, both hospitals used Kenny packs which consisted of steamed wool cloths wrapped around my upper arms, shoulders, back, chest, legs, and feet. The cloths were then wrapped in plastic to keep the heat in. I think I had those twice a day, and they were very hot.

We also had physical therapy which consisted of stretching for 10 minutes twice a day to keep our bodies mobile and prevent the tendency to tighten up. Tightening up causes deformation. Later, I remember hot wax treatments. They painted us with hot wax, and I remember a lot of the kids screamed over that. When the wax was pulled off, it took your hair off along with it.

I guess I spent a total of about two years at Sister Kenny. I even got my school lessons there. A tutor came in once a week to help me. I continued to get tutoring after I got out of the hospital, and I graduated from high school when I was 19.

The reason that they kept me at Sister Kenny for so long was that they thought I would improve enough that I wouldn't need the respirator anymore. The prevailing attitude, not from all the staff, but a lot of them, was that you weren't ever going to be worth anything if you remained in a respirator. That seemed to be the feeling, that you had to get out of the respirator to have any kind of a life. But by that time, I knew I was always going to need it.

Finally, the National Foundation started a policy of letting people take respirators home, so that's how I finally got to leave the hospital. I believe the Foundation owned them. They paid 40 or 50 dollars a week to either my parents or whomever my parents got to take care of me while I was at home. In addition to those payments, the National Foundation helped quite a bit with my hospital costs, which I'm sure were very high.

Later, my father worked for a gas company which had a huge insurance policy, so I was covered under that. It was hard when he retired, but by then Medical Assistance was starting to function. My parents took care of my grandmother who'd take care of me when they weren't home. After my father retired, he took care of my grandmother, and I'd hire people once in a while to go places with me. Then, when I was 14, I heard about Social Security disability. In order to apply for that I had to go to court to claim my independence and be adopted as a child of the court so that I could get benefits. From then on, I got a small income and used that to pay for things.

Though I was finally back home, my life had changed dramatically. Before I had polio, I was a very active child. I'd taken dance since I was three. I took ballet and tap dancing lessons. I was very strong. I guess I was really outgoing and extremely active from what my relatives tell me. I was constantly on the go. I remember my parents used to force me to lie down for naps every day. That drove me crazy. I wanted to be outside all the time.

I think my childhood was different than nowadays because my grandmother lived with us, and though my parents both worked, there was always someone at home with us, so I never had a babysitter or childcare. I was pretty much allowed to go where I wanted, when I wanted. I started cooking when I was five or six, and I used to cook everyone breakfast. I enjoyed food and needed a lot of it because I was so active. I had a lot of friends and would put on parades and plays and performances and force all my friends to come and watch.

But after I had polio, I think my friends changed. When I came home from the hospital, my old friends would come over to visit, but we just didn't have much in common. They seemed really childish to me. I guess I had left my childhood years behind and was an adult emotionally. I had dealt with issues like life and death, and I no longer had anything in common with my friends. They wanted to play, and I wasn't much interested in that. I still wanted to have friends my age, but it didn't work.

I did have one childhood friend whose friendship I maintained, and our parents were close, but mostly I just made new friends who were usually adults. We had more in common in dealing with adult issues. So I guess having polio resulted in the end of my childhood.

My relationship with my younger brother also changed somewhat. When I came back from the hospital, I wasn't the same big sister who used to play with him. When he brought his friends over, he would have to explain to them what all of the equipment was for and would demand that they say hello. I think also that after I came home he had a lot more responsibility. Yet, he seems to have dealt with it all very well.

I think I also handled it pretty well. It was something that happened, and I just dealt with it. I don't remember going through all the various stages that we are supposed to go through. I just accepted it. I think I was so busy dealing with life and death that I kind of skipped some of the stages and feelings I was supposed to have.

Anyway, I did get some continuing therapy after I came home, but it didn't help. I remember one therapist spent a lot of time working with my thumb, which was just kind of silly because none of my muscles worked except for some back muscles. I could just move the shoulder; nothing was going to help my thumb.

I also started to develop a scoliosis, and it has gotten much worse over the years. I lean to one side. Part of it's probably because I've chosen to use a wheelchair, and that caused me other problems too. Back in those days, wheelchairs did not recline, and I could sit only maybe an hour or so before my butt would really hurt. Eventually though, my father took a reclining lawn chair and put wheels on it. That was great. It solved the problem. After that, I could sit in the chair for a longer period of time before I had to go lie down.

That allowed me to get out more, but back then going out in public was quite difficult if you were in a wheelchair. I remember the first time I went out of the house and dealt with the so called "public" and how they perceived me. I think I had a pretty healthy outlook about myself, but we were walking down the street, and an old man came up and started walking ahead of me. He turned around and was walking backwards and started saying, "Oh you poor little girl," and I remember thinking, "Am I going to have to deal with this for the rest of my life? I don't want to." I think I started crying. When I got home, I went over to my bed in the dining room, which was a family problem in itself, and I was crying really hard, and both my mother and father said, "You're going to have to make a choice. Either live in the house without ever getting out to do things or else you can't let things like that affect you." My mother said I should've spit in his eye! So I just said, "The hell with it! I'm going out." And I did.

I'd like to say that was the last negative experience I had because of my wheelchair, but that wasn't the case. Discrimination against those of us who are in wheelchairs lasted a long time. I had a lot of problems with discrimination in the 1960's and 70's. I was asked to leave a restaurant, because it bothered the other customers, and I was asked to leave a concert at Northrup Auditorium. A friend of mine and I went to see this concert, and I was asked to leave because of an order by the fire marshall. I was ready to go up and ask the fire marshall (I always wanted to meet the man) if he really thought I shouldn't be there. I guess he figured I couldn't maneuver through the aisles very well, but I didn't think I was obstructing anything. Maybe he thought that in case of a fire people couldn't get out. It seemed to me that in case of a fire I'd be the one to get trampled. I was the one taking a chance. I left highly insulted.

In the same year, I went to see a friend's indoor marching band concert at the University, but that time I was not asked to leave. I don't know what the difference was between those two events. But back then, I was the only disabled person I ever saw going around town, so I guess they just didn't know how to react to me.

In 1970 I flew out to California to visit my brother. It was great because there were curb cuts everywhere. I could get into all the museums, and it was like this big revelation to me. I could do things I never considered doing in my own city because they simply weren't accessible. And when we drove over to L.A. to see some of our friends, it was like a whole new life for me. There were ramped places everywhere. So I thought about that a lot. I came home and thought about it some more. The civil rights movement had occurred ages ago. Well, not that many ages ago. I know it's still going on in some places, especially with racial injustice, but I realized that I'm part of it too. I live here too! I can vote if I choose to, but I can't get to a polling place because I can't get through the door. I have to get carried in, and have my wheelchair carried in. I never could use a public bathroom, and that wasn't right.

Then in 1974, I started hearing about how to connect with other people who were disabled. I don't even know how I heard about it, but I went to the first meeting, and there were some damned angry people there, people with the same frustrations as me. So I went to another meeting held at Augsburg College and attended a seminar given by Catholic Intervention Counseling. They were training us to be an organization and to fight the establishment using techniques and organizing tools. It was great.

I met a woman named Audrey, and she and I just clicked. She's a good organizer, and later she formed UHF (United Handicapped Federation). She held conventions and selected officers, all on her own. It was very good. I was able to be an officer and fit in as a member. It was a coalition of the various handicapped organizations; I think there were more than 20 at the time. We had this deep-down belief that we needed to organize, or we wouldn't be able to win. And we did accomplish a lot, but Audrey and I quit around 1979. By that time, it was beginning to turn into more of a social organization. I guess we accomplished enough things that people didn't see the same sense of urgency anymore.

About that same time, maybe 1979 or 1980, I had some really serious health problems. One morning my mother just couldn't wake me up, so she called the doctor, and I went into the hospital. I ended up having a tracheotomy. I spent about five months in the hospital, and when I got home there had been a big change. My mother was getting older, and she just wasn't able to carry me around anymore. She still did once in a while, but she was getting to the age where she shouldn't. My grandmother and my father had both died, so there was no one left to help with my care.

I realized that my mother just couldn't do it all herself anymore, so I decided to get personal care attendants. They wanted me to have somebody as a live-in, but I knew that the state paid people for only a few hours out of the 24, and that's not right. They'd be overworked, so I preferred to hire someone for every eight hours. The schedule goes from eight in the morning until four in the afternoon, and then four in the afternoon to midnight, and midnight to the next morning. The overnight shifts are pretty good for students. The trouble is, I stay up until about 12:30 A.M., so that makes it hard for them to study sometimes. I'm usually in the respirator during the evening though. At any rate, having the personal care attendants has worked out well for me.

I know my life would have been very different if I hadn't gotten polio, and though it's difficult to say what might have been, I guess I've always thought I would have been a dancer. Before I got polio, I danced all over. I was out of school half the year. My parents would take me to different programs to dance for various organizations. I remember once dancing at the Athletic Ball; they must've thought I was pretty good to have me dance for all those men. There were also a couple of ballets I auditioned for, and my mother said they wanted me to dance with their company. So I went over there to dance, but I was this eight-year-old snot. Driving home, my mother asked me what I thought of it, and I said, "Well, I didn't think they were very good." I felt relieved when my mother said I didn't have to dance there.

As I look back on it now, that was all I lived for, to dance. I remember asking for lessons at age three and if my mother would take me to a ballet, but then I got polio, and that ended my dance career. I don't even really know if I was any good, but I do know that I loved it, and I know that I danced all the time and that I was constantly on the go. Maybe, somehow, I was making up for all the time I was going to be held down.

David Kangas

In the fall of 1952, I was 15 years old and a sophomore in high school. I was a member of the football team and was looking forward to the start of basketball practice. The year before, I had been one of the few freshmen to make the varsity, so I had high hopes for the upcoming basketball season. However, the team had to get by without me because I developed polio on October third.

I suppose that my case was unusual in that I was the only one in my home town of Coleraine, Minnesota to develop polio that year. I did learn later that a woman from Coleraine had polio the year before. I think she was in her 20's, and if I remember correctly, there was another boy from the area who had it in 1953. But as far as I know, I was the only one out of the 500 students at my high school to have had polio in 1952.

I remember the day that I was diagnosed with polio very well. That morning, I was in physical education class at school, and we were out on the football field playing touch football. I noticed that as I was running, my leg would be weak, or sort of collapse under me. I didn't really think too much of it, but then later that day I was playing with the high school marching band at a polio benefit parade in Hibbing, which is about 30 miles from Coleraine where I grew up. During the march in that parade, my legs again became weak. In fact, they were so weak that I had to drop out of the line of march, and I went back to the school bus to lie down.

As part of the polio benefit that evening, there were stock car races. They were sending the proceeds from the races to the Polio Foundation. I was feeling pretty sick at that time, so I stayed in the school bus during the races whereas the other band members were out watching them. The band director came back to the bus, and after taking a look at me, he decided that he should find a car and drive me home. When I got home and my parents saw what condition I was in, they became very concerned. They called a doctor right away that evening. He came out to the house and made the diagnosis of polio and sent me to the Hibbing Hospital. I remember that I walked into the hospital, and that was the last time I was able to ambulate on my own.

After that, I had to be put in an iron lung for a few days. The Hibbing paper ran a picture of me in the iron lung, and the Duluth paper picked it up and also ran it. Believe it or not, a retired man from Duluth saw that picture and donated enough money to the Hibbing Hospital to buy another iron lung. He had been saving his money to buy a new car, but he said that the hospital needed the iron lung a lot more than he needed the car. I've still got a newspaper article about him and that incident.

Fortunately, I was able to breathe on my own again relatively quickly, so I only had to stay in the iron lung for about a week. However, the rest of my body didn't recover so well, and I was left with paralysis of both my lower extremities and my right arm and hand.

Once my condition was stabilized, I was given the Sister Kenny method of treatment with the hot packing. We called the women who came with the steamers and put the hot cloths on our legs and arms the "hot packers." They knew that it was uncomfortable, and they were always high spirited and joking and trying to keep our minds off of the pain and discomfort that we had to endure.

There happened to be two other fellows my age with polio at the Hibbing Hospital while I was there. After we felt well enough to get around in our wheelchairs, there was some comradery in that we were going through the same things, and also some high jinks. I remember we used to torment each other. If one was in bed and one was in a wheelchair, we would sort of play tricks on the guy in bed, knowing that he was virtually helpless. I remember one time one of the fellows somehow got some sticky materials that were used by the nurses and glued this other guy's toes together. Of course, he was screaming bloody murder about it, but he just couldn't move to defend himself. It was nothing malicious, but just the sort of tricks we played on each other.

I also remember that when I was at Hibbing Hospital, there was a visiting teacher who came to the hospital to give me my lessons so that I could keep up with my classmates. She actually was a "homebound teacher," and she got me through the rest of my sophomore year in high school.

However, I guess some of my most vivid memories from my time in the hospital are of the therapists who worked with us. They worked very hard on stretching the muscles to keep us limber and to reeducate some of the muscles that were still functional. They also taught us skills that we would need to maintain a level of independence.

I ended up staying at the Hibbing General Hospital from October until probably March, and then I transferred to the Sheltering Arms Hospital in Minneapolis, where I continued treatment until the end of the summer of 1953. When I was transferred down to Sheltering Arms, there was high anticipation that I was going to get some really great treatment. We had heard things about the whirlpool baths and some other treatments that we thought might help me, but I remember coming down with my parents and being quite disappointed. We asked, "Well, where are these whirlpool baths that we've heard about?" and we were shown the bathing rooms, and they just had a regular tub. The person said, "Well, whatever whirl you get is watching the water go down the drain." So, it was a big disappointment. Actually, the treatment at Sheltering Arms seemed to be more in terms of increasing your range of motion and getting you to realize that there wasn't any cure. Rather, you had to learn to get by with those muscles that were still working, and you had to start looking ahead to making a way for yourself as best you could.

I do remember one rather interesting event from my time at Sheltering Arms. A group of faith healers came to town, and some of the people at the hospital said, "We're going to the healing tent;

do you want to come along?" At that point I didn't care to go. Maybe I was too young. The guys who went were all in their 20's. I remember them coming back from the healing tent and telling us what happened. They said that the preacher had put his hands on them and told them to rise and walk. But, of course, they couldn't. They were still in their wheelchairs when they got back.

After about four months at Sheltering Arms, I realized that staying there was not really going to provide me with a cure. By that time I could see that I wasn't going to get any better. So one day I just said, "I want to see my doctor, and I want out of here. I want to go home, and I want to go back to school." I remember that the doctor didn't come until late that evening, and I had waited all day. When he finally came into my room, he sat down and asked, "Well, what do you want to do?" I told him exactly what I wanted to do. I told him that I didn't see any value in staying there any longer, and that I wanted to go home and just get on with my life. He wrote the discharge orders, and I left the next day.

Since I had spent a total of about 10 months in the hospital, I'm sure that the medical bills were huge, even back then in the 1950's. I wasn't too involved in our family finances, so I'm not sure of the amount or how it was paid, but I know my dad worked for the mining company. So there was insurance coverage for at least the hospitalization. I don't know how much they paid, but I'm sure they paid quite a good portion of it. The March of Dimes was also there to help pick up certain expenses. In fact, if I remember correctly, the local chapters could keep some of the money, and they also sent some to the National Foundation. As it turned out, our local chapter had more money than they could spend, so they would come around and say, "Do you need another new wheelchair, or can we get a ramp built to the house?" We did build a ramp, and the March of Dimes paid for it, so there was a lot of help with expenses.

I also remember distinctly that my dad was a Mason, and at Christmas of that first year, I remember him telling me that they had a Christmas gathering, and they had a benefit. They made sure that everyone there contributed, but they didn't say what it was for. When my dad came along, they encouraged him to put in a contribution, so he did. At the end of the celebration or gathering that night, they turned all the money over to my dad. I believe it amounted to several hundred dollars, and that was quite a bit back in those days.

I also was able to earn some money after I got out of the hospital. My home town of Coleraine always had a program of hiring some of the local kids to work in various jobs that the village had. I thought that there must be something I could do, so I approached the general maintenance foreman for the town and asked him if I could have a summer job. I was in a wheelchair, of course, so he asked, "Well, what do you think you can do?" I said, "You paint the curbs with the yellow markings, and you paint the parking areas; don't you? I can do that." He hired me, and that was my first job, painting the curbs in the town for that summer. I made a little money, and it really gave me a boost in terms of my self-esteem. In fact, I've still got a picture of me painting the streets in my wheelchair.

I went back to school that fall of 1953, and of course, back in those days, schools were not handicapped accessible. There were no elevators, so in order to get to the upper floors, a crew of several students would have to grab my chair and lift me up the steps. They did make some accommodations in the classroom itself, because they had to move desks around to fit my wheelchair in. There were also some arrangements made where I could stay for some classes on a lower floor, and the lessons would be brought down to me. A student monitor was there to help me, but for the most part, I was just carried up and down the steps.

I didn't like the idea of being dependent and having to rely on people to do this for me. However, I just had to face up to the fact that it was the only way I was going to get up to those other classes and continue on with my schooling. For the most part, the guys who helped me were quite willing to do it, but I sure didn't like it.

I remember the first time I went to a school function. I guess that I hadn't returned to school yet. I was still at Hibbing Hospital, so it would've been probably February or March when I came home from the hospital for a visit. I went up to the school to watch a basketball game. I very much wanted to do that because I had been on the basketball team the year before. I wasn't able to face up to seeing all those people at once, so I had it arranged to be lifted up the steps to a booth where I could watch the game. It was a projection booth, and enclosed, so people couldn't see me. However, word got around that I was there, and everybody was looking up and trying to catch a glimpse of me. It was kind of a tough hurdle for me to get over. But after the game, some people came up to talk to me as I was leaving the school. From that point on, I gradually became accustomed to having them see me as a disabled person, and I think that was the beginning of my acceptance of my disability.

I did have to have one surgery because of my polio. My hip

flexors had tightened up, so after my junior year of high school, I had an operation to correct that situation down at Gillette Hospital in Saint Paul. After that surgery, I was in a full body cast for about six weeks, so I missed part of my senior year, three months maybe. However, even with all the school I had missed, I was still able to graduate with my class.

After graduation, I got a job with the mining company as a posting clerk in the analysis laboratory. That was where they tested the ore. It was my job to record the analysis of the ore samples. I worked that summer, and the idea was, of course, that it was only summer employment. There was a junior college in the community up there, and it was the plan that I was going to attend the junior college. But September came, and the ore season wasn't over yet, so rather than quit and go to college, I continued on with the mining company until the end of the ore season, which was the end of November. I remember my parents were greatly concerned that I wasn't going to continue my education. I guess I just wasn't ready to go back to school yet, but I did start the winter quarter in January after I was laid off from the mining company. I started at the junior college, and then the next summer I went back to work for the mining company at the same job. I worked that whole summer, and then I came down to the University of Minnesota and started school that fall.

I met with the Vocational Rehabilitation Department, and it was their education plan for me to go to the University. I came down and looked around for an accessible apartment, which was almost impossible to find. I was really quite naive about going to college and was surprised to find that the University wasn't accessible for a person in a wheelchair. But that was 1955, and that's the way it was then. I saw that there were steps all over the place. It wasn't like high school where I had a group of friends to carry me around, but I still needed to find a crew of people to get me up and down the steps. Many times, I guess I could say many, I remember I would have to get a bunch of volunteers or just recruit people as they were rushing from class to class. Sometimes they would say, "I just don't have time. I can't help you," or they would say, "Well, I really have a bad back," which they may have had. So it was tough.

I remember that Ford Hall was the most difficult building, and I couldn't get into Northrup. I was able to get into Johnston Library pretty well, and some buildings had only one step, but Ford Hall was the worst. It had a split level entrance. There was an elevator, but you had to go up steps or down steps before you could get to the elevator. If I had to do it over again, I wouldn't have gone to the University. It took me five years to graduate because I had to drop so many classes. I just couldn't get to some classes enough because accessibility was such a problem.

I had to live in an apartment off campus because not one of the dorms was accessible. I found an apartment over by Loring Park, the Park Terrace Apartments, where you could drive into the building. It had inside parking. You could use the driveway into the garage, which was ground level, and so it was accessible for a wheelchair, and there were elevators in the building. Somehow, I had heard that there were several other people in wheelchairs who lived there. I ended up getting an efficiency apartment. It was a one-room efficiency, and the rent was $77 a month, unfurnished. I remember the Rehabilitation Department picked up $70 of that, so at least I got some financial help.

I also had my own car with hand controls, so I could drive from the apartment back and forth to the University. However, parking on campus was a real problem. There were no handicapped parking spaces. It was just a different time entirely. I had to find these sort of secret places where I could park without the University patrol coming along and ticketing me. I did have a disabled sign in the window, which sometimes helped. They never really gave me a ticket; they would just give me a warning. I remember there was one really good space behind the law building. There was this little nook in there, so I used to park there whenever I could.

I ended up getting an interdepartmental major that included courses in psychology, sociology, political science, and economics. I had started at the junior college in pre-engineering because, of course, my dad looked up to engineers. At the mining company, the engineer was the king. So that's why I started out in engineering, but when I got into the higher mathematics and physics, I could see those subjects were not my forte. So I came down to the University not really knowing what I wanted to study. Actually, it turned out that my strongest subjects were political science and sociology, and that eventually got me into my jobs in government.

While I was going to school and living at the apartment, I met Shirley, who is now my wife. We started dating, and when I graduated, which was after the winter quarter in 1960, I decided that I wanted to go out to California. I had some relatives in Sacramento, and I thought that rather than stay in Minnesota and deal with the winters here for the rest of my life, I would move out there. I graduated in March, and I asked Shirley to marry me and come with me out to California. She said yes, and we were married in April. On May 1, 1960, we packed up all of our worldly goods, which fit into the backseat and trunk of my 1957 Ford, and drove out to California.

We stayed at my aunt and uncle's home in Sacramento while we looked for a place to live, and I started looking for work. Shirley got a job with Aerojet General Corporation out there which was building the Polaris missile submarine or something like that. I took some civil service exams and got a job with the California Department of Motor Vehicles. We stayed there from May until the next January, which would have been January of 1961. However, we decided that we didn't like California after all, and we moved back to Minnesota.

When we came back here, at first I thought that maybe I should continue my education and pursue graduate studies, so I looked into the possibility of doing graduate work. I wrote to several colleges and universities. At the same time, however, I also took some civil service exams. I passed the exams and got several interviews. I remember one interview was for a job at the Minnesota State Prison. I went out to Stillwater and had the experience of hearing the iron doors clank behind me as I went through into the warden's office. My interview with the warden was for being a prison parole officer where I would make recommendations regarding prisoners who were eligible for parole. I didn't get that job, but I did end up getting a job as a research analyst with the State Department of Public Welfare. I began working there in March of 1961, and that sort of ended my formal academic training, although I did take some extension courses at the University. I worked with the state government for seven years and then transferred to Ramsey County, where I've been for the last 24 years.

Back in the 1960's, if you were disabled, just getting any type of job was a mammoth undertaking. If you could even get an interview, you were lucky. There was no affirmative action at all, and it quickly became apparent to me that in private industry, opportunities were virtually nonexistent. I recognized that the only reason I had gotten a job at the mining company was through my father being employed there, and they were just trying to do something to help our family. It wasn't a make-work job; it was a real job, but I wouldn't have gotten it if my dad didn't work there.

My first real job hunting was out in California, and I wrote letter upon letter, not getting any response. I couldn't even get an interview. I finally figured out that with civil service, if you took the exam and got the first, second, or third highest score, they would at least have to give you an interview. So that's what I did, and I had an interview with the Sacramento Municipal Utility District. Then I was in with the California Civil Service System, and that's how I eventually got the job with the Department of Motor Vehicles.

When we came back to Minnesota, I followed the same route. I took civil service exams, and I got the interviews. They could have still not hired me, because when I think about it, I was still competing with non-disabled people. But somehow, I managed to get the job.

Of course, there's been quite a change since those times. I think the job market is more open now to people with disabilities, although it's still quite competitive. I think at least part of that change is because of people who were forward enough or militant enough to say, "Look, in order for us to be independent, we need to have some accommodations made so that we have accessibility to the workplace." And finally, some of that has occurred.

There have also been some changes in people's attitudes toward the disabled. I think it's partly because there are more disabled people out there in the community now. You're no longer some oddity or freak. It's not just one person in a wheelchair. There are many wheelchair people. Years ago, someone in a wheelchair was a curiosity. Now, people are more used to seeing wheelchairs.

As far as my current situation, I'm still working full time, but over the last few years, I've been experiencing what is called post-polio syndrome. I'm weaker and just not able to do some of the things I was able to do five years ago. It takes me longer getting out of bed in the morning and getting ready to go to work. Also, I am finding that I have less stamina. I'm finding that I have to pace myself, and it's coming to the point now that I'll probably have to start working shorter days. I've got a lot of sick leave built up over the years, so maybe I'll just come home an hour early, or maybe it will get to the point where I'll be on an official part-time schedule. I'll just have to wait and see how it goes.

In 1990, I went to Sister Kenny Institute for a post-polio evaluation. Dr. Richard Owen did a number of tests to see where my muscle strength was at. He also evaluated my breathing because I was experiencing some problems there. I'll probably be going back pretty soon for a follow-up visit. I think it's good to have that sort of measurement to let you know where you're at. The studies have shown that maybe there's a one percent per year loss in strength, so you have to be prepared and deal with it.

From time to time, of course, I have thought about what my life might have been like without polio. I was quite active in sports before I had polio. Like I said, I was on the football team when I came down with it. My sport was really basketball though, and I was really looking forward to the coming season. However, I came down with polio in October which was before the season started. So I feel I probably would have had at least a high school career in sports, and maybe a college career as well.

I was also interested in music, and I had thought about maybe being a musician. But after polio, with the decrease in breathing and my lungs, I could still play, but I don't think I could have been a professional musician. However, I actually played in high school and college dance band even after polio. I played the cornet, with the three valves.

It's interesting; there's a little anecdote in terms of involvement with polio where you overuse something during the critical stage when you're first coming down with the disease. Well, the day I was diagnosed, I had played my coronet in the polio benefit up in Hibbing. I think playing the coronet was part of the reason my right hand was so severely affected. After polio, I had to switch and play my instrument with my left hand. I also had to switch and learn how to write left-handed, which was quite a challenge since I was right-handed, but I did it.

I think these are some things that would have been different if I didn't have polio. It's also very likely that I would have had a different career. But, who knows? And I really can't complain. My life has been good in spite of having polio.

Chapter 4

Under the Knife

Many of those we interviewed underwent surgical procedures because of their polio. Most often, these were operations on their legs and feet. The three women whose interviews are included in this chapter had a total of 16 surgeries between them. Their stories seem to capture the essence of the surgical experience all too well.

Kay Brutger

In 1950 when I was nine months old, my mother took me to the doctor to get vaccinated for diphtheria, tetanus, and whooping cough. That very night I came down with polio. My mom tells me she was changing my diaper, and I just started to scream. She also noticed that my one leg dropped down, and I couldn't lift it up. Mom and dad knew that something was wrong, so they called the doctor. He told them to bring me into his office, and after examining me, he said, "We'll have to admit her to the hospital. It looks like she has polio." So I went into the hospital, and they confirmed the diagnosis.

My mom tells me that I was in isolation for a while, and I guess I spent a total of about two or three months in the hospital. After getting out of isolation, I got the treatment with hot packs as well as some other types of therapy, though I don't think any of it really helped very much. I think that my mom stayed at the hospital with me the whole time I was there.

I got out of the hospital some time in December and was home for Christmas. My parents had to do exercises with me because I was left with paralysis in my right leg and hip. Due to the paralysis, I didn't start to walk until I was about 18 months old, and I was put in a leg brace about that same time. The brace went from my ankle to my knee and helped to support me when I walked. I guess I wore that until I was six years old.

I don't really remember that much about my early childhood, though my mom tells me that I missed out on a lot of things. I couldn't run and play like the other kids, so my mom says that I was deprived of a normal childhood.

As I grew, my legs became increasingly asymmetrical. My left leg was normal, but my right leg was skinny and weak. My right foot didn't work very well. It was what they used to call a "drop foot." They also diagnosed me as having osteoporosis in that foot. So when I was six, I had the first of my four surgeries.

I do have some clear memories about that surgery. I remember that my parents took me to Minneapolis the night before I went into the hospital. We stayed at a hotel, and I had to sleep in a crib. Being six years old, I recall feeling quite embarrassed about having to sleep in that crib.

The next morning, my parents took me to the hospital. They left me there with the nurses, and if I close my eyes, I can still see them walking down the hall and getting on the elevator. Being separated from my parents for the first time (at least the first time I can remember) made me feel very lonely and frightened. Since we lived about two hours away, my mom stayed down in the Twin Cities while I was hospitalized. I'm very thankful for that. She stayed with a friend who lived in Minneapolis, and every day during the two weeks or so that I was there, she took a cab to the hospital to visit me.

The surgery involved putting a plate in my right leg, an ivory "screw" in my right knee, and attaching an artificial cord up over the top of my right foot. I remember that after the surgery, I was put on a ward with a lot of other children. My leg had to be elevated, and it seemed to me that every time a visitor, doctor, or nurse came through that ward, they would bump that leg. And oh, it hurt!

I also remember that getting the stitches out was quite an ordeal. Back in those days, the stitches were made of cat gut. The doctor would rub them down with alcohol as hard as he could in order to loosen them up. Then he would cut them and pull them out. Well, I had seven incisions for that surgery and well over 100 stitches. So getting them out took a lot of rubbing and pulling. It was a gruesome and painful experience. My dad couldn't watch. It made him so sick that he had to leave the room. Thank goodness that my mom was able to stay in the room with me until the bitter end.

Though I guess the surgery was successful, my foot is still as flat as a pancake, and it's still a drop foot. However, I didn't have any pain with that foot for many years, and I'm certainly thankful for that. Recently, though, I've started to have pain in my hip and lower back. I guess that limping for all those years has started to catch up with me.

When I got out of the hospital, I was still wearing a cast, so my mom had to deliver me to and from school in a baby buggy. Needless to say, that was quite embarrassing. I had to use crutches to get around the school, and that wasn't always easy. Of course, nothing was handicapped accessible back in those days, not even in a school.

I don't remember having any therapy after that first surgery. However, I do know that I had to wear a leg brace and a built-up shoe for a while. That brace and shoe were very cumbersome to drag around all day.

In spite of that brace and built-up shoe, I did most of the things the other kids did. I jumped rope, played baseball, even ice skated. I wasn't particularly good at all the things that I tried, but I was able to do most anything the other children did, as long as it didn't involve running or climbing trees. The kids never made fun of me and generally included me in what they were doing.

I don't think that I was babied by my parents or treated any differently than my brothers and sister. Except for getting polio, I was always a healthy child. However, I tired more easily than my siblings. Still, I had chores to do. I helped with the housework and weeded the garden just like everybody else.

Fortunately, my dad worked for the Great Northern Railroad, and so we had hospitalization coverage. That paid for most of my hospitalization and surgeries, but my parents had to pay for everything else such as therapy, crutches, wheelchairs, braces, and outpatient services. I am very grateful to them for everything that they did. I know that I can never repay them. Our family was certainly not wealthy, and we stretched every dollar. And believe me, I was a very expensive child. Not only did I have polio, but I also needed braces on my teeth and new eyeglasses every year. So, I know that I must have been quite a financial burden for my parents.

I had my second surgery when I was 11. My right leg wasn't growing as fast as the left one, so they operated on my left leg to slow its growth so that there wouldn't be such a large disparity between the two. They did this by putting staples in the knee area. During that same surgery, they also operated on my left foot. That foot sort of turned in when I walked, so I would walk on the side of it. The surgeon tried to turn it back the way it was supposed to be.

For some reason, I really don't remember anything about that surgery or my subsequent stay in the hospital. I do know that I had a lot of trouble with a "trick knee" after the surgery. The kneecap would just sort of snap out of place when I walked. I'm not sure why that would happen, but six years later in 1967, when I was 17, I had my third surgery to try to correct that problem. During this third surgery, they put eight screws and two plates in my knee and thigh. The incision was in the same place as the one from the previous surgery. It extended along the whole length of the thigh.

When I woke up after that surgery, I found myself in a body cast that extended from my shoulders all the way down to my left foot. Only my right leg and foot weren't covered by the cast. Before the surgery, no one had told me that I'd be in such a huge cast, and when I saw it, I remember being so depressed that all I could do was cry.

I went home from the hospital in that cast and wore it for the next six months. All I could do was lie in one position, flat on my back. My parents had to bring me home in a station wagon on a stretcher that was borrowed from the fire department. We had to rent a hospital bed and set it up in the living room because that was the only place in our house where the bed would fit. The cast was so heavy that I couldn't turn over by myself. If I wanted to change position, my mom had to turn me and then prop pillows under me so I wouldn't roll back. I know that I disturbed her sleep many a night just so that I could be repositioned. I couldn't attend school, of course, so a teacher had to come to the house and bring me my lessons. I couldn't sit up and had to do all my school work lying down.

When the cast finally came off, I thought that things would get back to normal, and I'd be able to get on with my life. Unfortunately, that wasn't the case. Instead, I had to return to the hospital for about a month so I could receive extensive physical therapy. I also found out that a mistake had been made when they put me in the cast. They had set my left foot at the wrong angle, and after being like that for six months, it stayed that way. They tried to stretch the foot back into place with weights but were unsuccessful. They also were supposed to have inserted little sponges at the pressure points, such as the heel and by the little toe. Because they hadn't inserted those sponges, when the cast came off, a lot of skin and meat came off with it!

Because of that surgery, I am no longer able to wear high heels or ice skates. The foot and ankle are just too weak. Even though the surgery was performed more than 25 years ago, I still suffer from its effects. I have trouble walking, and I get a very painful callous on my foot. I should go to the doctor once a month to have the callous removed, but it's expensive to have it done. So I take care of it on my own and put off going to the doctor until the pain is unbearable.

After several months of trips back and forth to the hospital for therapy, I was finally able to go back to high school. Since there was no such thing as a handicapped accessible school bus, I had to commute to school by taxi cab. After school, the taxi would take me to the hospital for a couple hours of therapy. My dad would then have to pick me up from the hospital and bring me home for supper and homework. It wasn't what I had anticipated my senior year of high school would be like, but my stubbornness and strong-willed nature got me through all the long, tedious hours of therapy. Not only did I learn to walk again, but I graduated with my class that June as an honor student.

I had my fourth, and hopefully last surgery when I was 35 years old. At that time, my "good" leg, which is my left leg and on which I already had two surgeries, was throbbing with pain. I first thought it was arthritis, so I just put up with the pain until it became unbearable. I went back to the clinic in Minneapolis where they had my old records, but I found out that the physician who had done my previous surgeries was no longer in practice. Therefore, I had to schedule an appointment with a new doctor who knew nothing about my case.

The new doctor to whom I was referred said that I needed another surgery to find out why I was having such extreme pain. So I went back into the hospital, and they opened up that left leg again. They went through the same incision that they had made during my last surgery in 1967. The doctor ended up taking out all the old screws and plates. He also realigned the kneecap, which apparently had not been positioned correctly during the previous surgery. While they were in there, they found a lot of scar tissue, which was apparently the source of my pain, so they cut out as much of that as they could. The doctor also used arthroscopic surgery to repair the cartilage and ligaments around the knee. So it ended up being quite an extensive surgery.

When I came out of the anesthetic, I was expecting to really feel miserable, but I found out that surgery has come a long way since 1967. I actually felt well enough to sit up and eat supper just a couple of hours after waking up. The next day they put the leg on a machine that kept my knee in motion 24 hours a day. That was to keep the scar tissue from growing back again. Each day they changed the angle at which the knee was bent until it reached 90 degrees. After that, I got some additional therapy for range of motion in the knee and leg.

Though that surgery helped reduce my leg pain, when I was about 40, my back started to really bother me. I could still put in a 10 hour day at work, but when five o'clock rolled around and I went home, I didn't have the strength to make supper or do the dishes. So I went to an orthopedic surgeon here in Bowling Green, Kentucky. I gave him all my old records; he studied them, took some x-rays, and discovered that after all these years of walking with a limp, I have worn down two small bones on either side of the vertebrae in my back. That problem, along with arthritis in that area, is what was causing my back pain. To help alleviate the problem, I now wear a leg and foot brace. The brace is made of lightweight plastic and goes under my foot and in back of my leg. It is secured with a velcro strap under the knee. It holds up my "drop foot" so that I don't have to lift it up so high when I walk. I don't limp as badly anymore. For the $350 that it cost, you'd think it was made out of gold! But actually, I should have had this type of brace 20 years ago.

The brace has helped my back pain, though it still bothers me sometimes. When it does, I do back exercises. I also ride a stationary bike for exercise, but I avoid doing too much walking because of the callous on the bottom of my foot. I also have poor circulation in my right leg. It turns numb, and it's usually purple in color. I believe that all these problems are due to that one surgery that I had. But I feel pretty good 99% of the time. If I could just get rid of that spot on the bottom of my foot, I'd be in good shape.

As far as other aspects of my life, I've been married to the same man since 1971 and have two beautiful daughters, born in 1974 and 1978. They are both healthy and have strong, beautiful legs. I don't think that polio has limited me too seriously. I'm too stubborn to let it! I enjoy country western music and love to go dancing. Though I often feel tired and sore the next day, I'm not about to give up dancing. I enjoy gardening and have a nice-sized garden. I love flowers and shrubs, so weeding keeps me busy. I go motorcycle riding and swimming, and I love to cook and sew. All of these activities have gotten harder for me over the years, but I keep on trucking because I don't enjoy sitting around.

I have worked at various factory jobs most of my life, and somewhere along the way, I got into optics. I worked my way up, and eventually became a supervisor. When we moved to Bowling Green, Kentucky in 1988, I got a job in a bank and worked there for several years. However, the bank downsized, and I had to look for another job. I was fortunate enough to find a wonderful job as a consultant for a regional sewer system. I handle the grant money paperwork for projects that deal with the Environmental Protection Agency, and I enjoy my work very much.

I think that I have a nice personality and a pretty face, and perhaps that's why I've been fairly well accepted wherever I went. Making new friends has always been difficult for me, however, because I always wonder how they are going to react to someone who limps and has two of the ugliest legs in town. I guess I've always been afraid that they will reject me.

Though my experiences with polio may have resulted in me developing a kind heart and learning the importance of patience, I've often wondered what my life would have been like if I hadn't had polio. Because I've been in and out of hospitals all of my life, I believe that I'm a different person than I would have been if I wouldn't have had polio. I'm bitter sometimes, but I know that there are people out there who are in a lot worse shape. So the bitterness quickly passes. Still, I wonder what it would have been like to be normal and have two healthy legs. I can't help but think that I would have had one hell of a good time!

Gail Bias

I was born in 1949 and was raised on a farm in rural St. Wendel, Minnesota. Maybe because I have a twin brother and we did so many things together, I was quite a tomboy when I was a child. However, I was diagnosed with polio in August of 1951 when I was two years old. Because of that illness, my childhood ended up being quite different than my brother's.

Since I was so young when I had it, I don't remember anything about the actual disease. In fact, I really don't have a lot of memories about my early childhood. Some people can remember things from when they were one or two. I can't do that. I do remember that when I was little, I used to think that I got polio from playing in the grease by the garage. Now, what would make a child think that, I don't know. Maybe that was one of the stories going around back then about how people got it. Who knows?

Anyway, my mother has told me that the day I came down with polio, she came into my room to get me up from my nap. When she tried to pick me up, I started to scream. Every time she tried to touch me I would just scream. The epidemic was very bad that year, so my mom tells me that she knew right away that I had polio. She called the doctor, and I was then admitted to St. Cloud Hospital.

My hospital records show that I was put in isolation for 18 days, but I don't remember any of it. I guess my earliest memories having to do with polio start at about the age of five and relate to my visits to Gillette Hospital where they did my reconstructive surgeries. I remember going down this long, dark corridor at Gillette. I can picture myself wearing leg braces and using my walking sticks to help me walk. Darkness always seemed to be a part of that place, at least in my memories. And believe me, these are not happy memories. It seems to me that I cried constantly every time I was there.

I probably didn't have my first surgery until I was about six years old. Up until then, I think my visits to Gillette were just to get my braces fitted. But when I was six, I had my first reconstructive surgery. It was a very lonely time for me. I remember that I could only have visitors from two to four on Saturday and Sunday, and with farm chores, the only day my mom and dad could come was Sunday. I'd cry while I was waiting for them to arrive; I'd cry the whole time they were there; and then I'd cry after they left. It was such an empty, empty feeling, being there all alone. I didn't really know my roommate, and she probably was feeling as badly as I was. So she couldn't have comforted me anyway.

I remember that after your surgery, they would write on your cast what kind of a procedure they had done. It was kind of their trademark. Also, there were a lot of interns from the University of Minnesota there, and that way when an intern or somebody came around to examine you, they'd know what was done. It was rather impersonal, I always thought, to identify you by your surgery. But that's the way they did it back then.

I have really vivid memories of that stay in the hospital and that first surgery. I remember getting scrubbed with antiseptic the evening before my surgery. They had these huge, metal tubs, and you had to climb up steps to get in them. And when you were done, they laid towels on the steps and on the floor all the way to your bed for you to walk on so your feet wouldn't touch the floor. Once you got back in bed, you weren't supposed to get up again until your surgery. Then at midnight, they'd come into your room, wake you up, and put this red vest on you. That red vest meant that you were all prepared for surgery. They'd actually tie it on, so you couldn't take it off. Of all the colors, I've often wondered why in the world they chose red!

You never really knew what was going on. I don't think that I even knew what that first surgery was for. They didn't tell you, and you didn't dare ask. At least I didn't. But, the more surgeries I had, the more I got accustomed to the routine and what was going to happen. I have all these cruddy memories of my surgeries, and they all sort of blend together.

Of course, I could never sleep the night before any of my surgeries. It was always early morning by the time I'd fall asleep. Then you'd hear the cart coming down the corridor. You'd hope the cart was coming for someone else, and if it would go past your door, you'd breathe a little bit easier. But then your door would fly open, and you knew the cart was there for you. It was your turn. And then you just got on the cart. You didn't fuss. You'd just look up at the lights whizzing by as they pushed the cart down the hall and into the operating room.

I remember that the operating room was always cold. And you'd have to crawl off of the cart onto that cold operating table. Then they'd put these big, leather straps over your leg and tighten them up. I guess that was to cut the flow of blood when they operated, but I remember lying there terrified and thinking that they were going to cut me open, and I wasn't even asleep yet. The nurses would try to comfort you, but it really didn't help. And by that time, you couldn't even cry any more because of all the medication they had given you.

I think the only thing that got me through all those surgeries was knowing that when I woke up, my mom would be there. Mom was always there for me. If the surgery was at 6:00 A.M., mom would be there by nine or so when I woke up. Knowing she'd be there was a tremendous comfort for me.

Surgeries were always on Monday. At least that was the day my doctor did surgery. And it was always early in the morning. I had a total of six surgeries, and the schedule never changed. They were always on Monday morning, and I got so that I knew the routine very well. I eventually knew just what to expect.

I guess I had my second operation when I was about 10. During that surgery, they transplanted my heel cord to the front of my foot because that foot was what they called a "drop foot." I couldn't raise the foot at all. The brace on my shoe would hold it, but they wanted to try this experimental surgery, so they transplanted the heel cord. Mine was one of the few that was successful, and I do have some motion in that foot. So many of those surgeries either didn't work or resulted in bad infections. I was very fortunate to have had six surgeries and to never have one result in an infection.

I had my third surgery about one year after the second one. It was a reconstructive surgery where they broke all the bones in my left foot and reconstructed it to be more like a normal foot. When I came out of the anesthetic, I had all these rods that held the bones together sticking out of my foot. It was very painful, but I was excited about that surgery because I thought it was going to fix my foot so that I'd be like everybody else. I remember the kids in school used to laugh at me, so it was very important to me that I get that foot reconstructed.

Two weeks after that, I had yet another surgery. That one was on my right leg. It involved a "bone block" to stop that leg from growing. That way there wouldn't be such a big difference between my two legs.

I guess I was in the hospital for a total of about two months for those two surgeries. I even had my school lessons there, so I didn't fall too far behind. I missed my regular school, but I had nice teachers at the hospital, so it wasn't that bad.

I remember that after I got to feeling better, I was moved into a ward with all these other girls, and eventually, I developed some friendships. I remember that we'd get in these old wooden wheelchairs like they used to have back then, and we'd race down the hall as far as we could go. Sometimes if we wanted to make a little noise, we'd throw ice out of the ice machine at the end of the hall, and of course, we'd catch hell for that. But we were just kids trying to make the best of our situation and have a little fun.

Holidays were always the hardest time to be in the hospital, and though I was never there over Christmas, I did have to spend one Easter in the hospital. If somebody brought you something good to eat when you were on the ward, you were expected to share it with everybody, and it would be given out at 2:00 P.M. with orange juice. But if your mom brought candy, you didn't always want to share it because there probably wasn't enough for all 25 or so of the girls on the ward. So when my mom brought me candy at Easter, I hid it in my bed pan! That seemed like the safest place to put it. After all, who in the world would ever go looking for something to eat in a person's bed pan?

I also remember that after those two surgeries, I wanted to go home very badly. But I had casts on both legs, and my right knee had to be totally immobilized for quite a while. I remember begging the doctor to let me go home, but he thought I should stay. Well, one day he came into the ward where I was staying with all these other girls, and like usual, I started begging him to let me go home. So he said, "Well now, how about if I give you some crutches, and we'll see how you do with them." They got me some crutches, and I took off and went across the room and back, and then I said, "Now can I go home?" Well, he looked at the nurses and said, "Send this girl home. She'll probably fall down like a turtle, but I'll be damned if she won't get back up and get going again." So even though I still had those two casts on my legs, I got to go home. And really, I did just fine.

Of course, I had to go back periodically for check-ups, and I always dreaded that. It seemed like those examinations were always the same. We'd always take the same route down to Minneapolis, and after we got there, I'd have to go to this dressing room that was sort of like a high school gym locker room and get undressed. They'd always give me this little loin cloth, something like a diaper, to put on. It had strings at both ends, and you'd tie it around your waist, and then they'd put this hospital gown over you. Then you'd go into a little cubicle and sit on this wooden table, and the whole room would be full of doctors. There'd be interns in there, and of course, your surgeon, and somebody to take notes, and they'd touch you, and probe you, and bend you like you were some sort of scientific specimen. After that, you'd go to x-ray, and then physical therapy. You'd go here and there, and the day was very grueling for a young child. I always dreaded going down there, but they treated everybody the same, and you had no choice but to go down there and go through it.

After I had my reconstructive surgeries, I didn't need to wear braces anymore, just a built-up shoe. But school was still hard for me, not academically, but socially. I went to a one-room schoolhouse, and even though I knew everyone there, it was very difficult to be the only child in the school with a disability. I still had a very noticeable limp, and the other kids used to make fun of me, but after a while, they accepted me pretty well. I guess they got used to me. I was even included when they played ball at recess. I couldn't run, but they let me play anyway.

Going to high school was particularly difficult for me. It was such an adjustment to go from a one-room, country school where you knew everybody to the high school in town. I had two strikes against me. First of all, I was a country kid, and the kids from town used to tease me about that, but I also wore a built-up shoe and walked with a limp, so I got made fun of quite a bit.

Being different is really hard when you're in high school. I ended up just not participating in a lot of things that I probably would have participated in if it wasn't for my disability. I would have liked to try out for cheerleading, but people made fun of me just for talking about it. So I ended up keeping a lot of feelings inside. I didn't want to go to a dance because I was self-conscious of my limp. I didn't want to have people stare at me as I walked across the dance floor. I hated to have people gawk and laugh at me. I think all teenagers are self-conscious, but when you have some physical disability, it really magnifies that self-consciousness. To this day, I hate it when people stare at my leg when I wear shorts. But I'll be damned if I'm going to let that stop me from wearing shorts, because I like to wear them. People are curious, of course, so it's only natural to look, but they don't have to stare. When somebody stares at me, I'll turn around and stare back at them. It may be rude, but perhaps it will teach them not to gawk at people with disabilities.

I end up wearing long skirts and boots a lot, so people don't notice my legs. It's interesting, but I think people accept me much better if they meet me when I'm seated at a table, and they don't know anything about my disability. When people see me walk and notice my limp, they are much more likely to be stand-offish. I've had that happen many, many times, so I know it's not just all in my imagination.

Anyway, getting back to my experiences during childhood and adolescence, I was never treated any differently by my parents or other members of my family. I was never excluded. I suppose I was very lucky in that I had excellent family support. I did chores on the farm. I didn't bale hay, but I drove the tractor, and I did virtually everything else, or at least I tried to do everything else. One thing that's kind of interesting though, is that I guess I always thought I had to prove myself by keeping up, so I never gave up; I never said, "I can't do that." The hardest thing in the world for me was to say,

"I can't." I'm not sure if I was trying to prove myself to other people or to myself, but I think I kind of burned myself out doing that. There are a lot of things that I just can't do. I can't skip; I can't stand on one leg, but I'd never admit to anyone that I couldn't do those things. I remember in physical education classes, I would just sort of try to blend into the back of the class. It took me a long time, but now I'm finally able to say, "I can't." Now if someone is walking too fast for me to keep up, I'm able to say, "Go ahead. I'll catch up with you later." For most of my life, I couldn't do that. It's a shame that you get smart so late in life!

As far as more recent experiences, I had another surgery about nine years ago. That surgery was done at Abbott Northwestern Hospital. I was referred there by my doctor at Sister Kenny Institute. In that surgery, they opened up my foot, and I thought they were going to correct my "hammer-head heel," but they didn't. What's worse is that I had some severe problems after that surgery. The stitches broke, and the heel pad came loose. I can actually grab it and move it. So I tried to see the surgeon who had done the operation, but he wouldn't see me. He was gone on "sabbatical." I ended up having to see one of his colleagues, and he opened it back up, and it was awful. The surgery probably never should have been done in the first place. It took about six months to heal, but I can walk barefooted at least a little bit now, so it wasn't a total loss. However, I still have a lot of problems with my feet. The "hammer-head heel" is still there, and my big toe was fused incorrectly, so it's crooked. I've had a bunion removed, and I need two different size shoes, so buying shoes is always a nightmare.

In addition to the problems with my feet, over the last several years or so, I've been having other polio-related problems. I get fatigued very easily, and some of my muscles have gotten weaker. I went down to Sister Kenny Institute to get my situation evaluated, and the doctor there told me that the nerve cells that were affected by polio had originally regained some of their strength, but now, years later, those nerve cells are just dying. So I can't do some of the things that I used to be able to do. For instance, I can't stand to swim anymore, and I have trouble breathing if there's any pressure on my chest. I can't sleep if I'm lying on my left side because that makes it hard for me to breathe. I also have weakness in my hands, and I have some problems with bladder control.

I was put on a medication for the fatigue, but it just didn't seem to do any good. So the doctor put me on a low dosage of Ritalin. I'm not a medication taker by nature because when I had my surgeries as a child I became addicted to the painkillers they had given me, and the withdrawal was very painful. So I was hesitant to take a medication that might be addictive. I was told to take the Ritalin only if I felt that my energy was really low, so I only took it once in a while when I was really suffering. It did work; it'll work on anybody, but the doctors decided that Ritalin wasn't the right medication for me, so I don't take it anymore.

The doctor at Sister Kenny also recommended that I ride a stationary bike for exercise and to help reduce my fatigue. So I spent $500 on this bike and went on their exercise program. I was supposed to ride the bike 15 minutes and then rest for 5 minutes, and then do 15 more minutes on the bike. I tried it for two weeks, but I kept getting weaker. When I'd get off the bike, I'd have to lie down on the floor because I couldn't use my left leg. I'd get off the bike and fall flat on my face until my leg started to work again. I was destroying what I was trying to build up, so I stopped riding the bike.

When I went back down to Sister Kenny Institute for a follow-up evaluation, and the doctor asked me how my exercise program was going, I told him I wasn't doing it. I told him what had happened and that I couldn't even walk after riding the bike. The doctor got really upset and said, "Well, why the hell wasn't somebody doing some follow-up." I told him that no one had called me, and I was so angry about the whole thing that they just sent me home. So I really haven't gotten much help for my post-polio problems.

I've often wondered what my life would have been like if I wouldn't have had polio, but it's hard for me to imagine. I have basically been like this all of my life, or at least as long as I can remember, so I have nothing to compare it to. I don't know what it would be like to be able to run, and that bothers me sometimes. I would love to be able to jog or play tennis. I'm a farm girl, and I'm an outdoors-type person at heart. But I'm not physically fit enough to do a lot of the things that I would like to do, and sometimes that makes me mad because I never had the chance to try so many things.

There is one benefit that came out of my having had polio, however. I find that handicapped people, especially children, seem to relate to me very well. There's just sort of a natural connection there, and in my work as a social worker, that can be very helpful. On balance though, certainly the negative effects of polio far outweigh any benefits. Yet, I try not to dwell on the negatives because I think I've made the best of my situation.

Barb Johnson

I had polio at the age of three. Since I was so young then, I really don't remember anything about my initial illness, but my mom has told me that I started to develop a temperature on Saturday, October 10, 1959. By Sunday, I started to fall down when I'd try to walk, and then on Monday, my neck was stiff and sore. My mom called the doctor, and he just told her to watch me, but later that day, the doctor told my mom to bring me in to see him. I'm not sure exactly what happened after that, but I was diagnosed with polio that day and ended up at Sister Kenny Institute in Minneapolis.

When we got to Sister Kenny, my mom says that they made me walk and then run down the hallway to see if I would fall. Apparently, they thought I might just be faking it to get attention. My mom says that made me very angry. I guess they couldn't believe that I had polio because I had been vaccinated and even had all of my booster shots.

After the doctor realized that I wasn't faking, I was admitted to the hospital and put into isolation. The next day my mom came to visit me, but they wouldn't allow her in my room, not that she hadn't already been exposed! After about three weeks, I was moved to a ward with 15 other kids. There were eight of us on each side of the ward, and a curtain ran down the middle. We were all three years old or younger, and according to my mom, I was the only one on the ward who'd been vaccinated.

My mom recalls that there were kids on that ward from all over the country. Since some were from so far away, their parents couldn't be there very often. My parents were there all the time, so some of the other kids called them "mom and dad." I thought that was pretty neat. I don't remember much else, though. I can recall people in white coats and a certain smell, sort of like a hot, catalytic converter. I assume that was the smell from the hot packs that they wrapped us in.

I mostly remember that I wasn't very happy. My mom has a picture of me sitting in my hospital bed with a tray full of mashed potatoes in front of me. I have a strange look on my face, and it's certainly not a happy look. After all, I was three years old and in the hospital with polio. There wasn't much to be happy about. I don't think my siblings were very happy either. There are five children in my family; I'm the youngest. I think my siblings really missed my parents a lot. Not only were my parents gone when I first had polio, but they were also gone for my surgeries. So I'm sure that was very difficult for them.

I was in the hospital until about the middle of January. After I was home, I remember going back to Sister Kenny to see Dr. Richard Owen. I don't remember any specific trips, but I know I went to see him for many years.

When I first got out of the hospital, I was still using Kenny sticks to walk. They were just little wooden sticks with leather bands on the end that went around your arm. However, I must have gotten off of them pretty quickly, because I remember an incident that occurred when I was very young. My mom heard about a girl who needed my Kenny sticks, so we met her family in a parking lot somewhere and gave them the sticks. I have no idea why we met them in that parking lot, but I remember being very happy about giving those sticks to someone who could use them.

I know that I was off of the Kenny sticks sometime before I started school, and I never needed braces. However, I did end up having six surgeries on my legs and feet. Of course, I had to use crutches to get around for a few weeks after each surgery. In fact, during kindergarten I was on crutches, not the Kenny sticks, but regular crutches, so I must have had my first surgery when I was five. I'm not sure what they did during that surgery, but I know I had scars on the sides of my feet after the bandages came off.

I remember that I missed some kindergarten because of that first surgery. When I came back to school, the boys used to steal my crutches and play machine gun with them. The teacher would have to get them back for me. I also remember that they wanted to put me in special education, and it wasn't special education for kids with physical handicaps. I would have been segregated off into a classroom with mentally handicapped children. I guess they thought that since I was physically handicapped, I must be mentally handicapped as well. Fortunately, my parents wouldn't allow it, and I'm very thankful for that.

Actually, I seemed to fit in quite well in my kindergarten class. I did virtually everything the other kids did. However, one thing that I couldn't do was skip. I could only gallop, so that year, instead of learning how to skip, all the kids in my class learned how to gallop. That way, I wouldn't feel left out. So I think I had a pretty good kindergarten teacher.

I didn't have my next surgery until I was about 10, so my elementary school years were pretty normal. I got my share of teasing and stuff, but typically it was short-lived, and I had other kids who would stick up for me. I lived in sort of a rural area, and I went to the same small school throughout my elementary years. The kids all knew me, and that helped a lot. Outside of my little network of school and neighborhood, other kids that I didn't know would sometimes make fun of me, but I learned to just ignore it and go forward. Maybe I'd cry after I got home, but I'd be tough when it happened and wouldn't let them know how much it hurt.

To tell you the truth, I think that I had a pretty good childhood. I did almost everything that the other kids did. I climbed trees, played baseball, and swam. I think that I spent more time outside than my kids do now. The one thing that I didn't do, not until I was 11, was ride a bike. The doctors said I shouldn't try to ride a bike, but when I was 11, I finally got the okay to have one. My dad took me outside and pushed me around until I figured out how to ride it. I was the only one in my family to get a brand new bike. Everyone else got hand-me-downs, but mine had a gearshift and hand brakes. It was pretty cool!

The five year break between my first and second surgeries ended when I was 10. From then on, I had surgery about every other summer for the next several years. All my surgeries were done at Mayo Clinic in Rochester, and they were all performed in late August. Each time, I was probably in the hospital for about two weeks, and then I went home in time to start school. I would still be on crutches when school started, but by scheduling my surgeries at the end of August, I didn't miss out on too much of the summer. I liked it that way.

Since I had so many surgeries, they all sort of blend together in my memory. A couple of incidents do stick in my mind, though. I don't remember during which surgery this happened, but after one of the operations, the first thing I said when I came out of the anesthetic was, "I'm not crying, mom!" I guess I was trying to be brave for my mother. I was expected to be brave and tough. Maybe my mom even told me not to cry. I don't know, but that's the first thing I said when I woke up.

I also remember being on a ward with a young man who had been wounded in Viet Nam, so that must have been during one of my later surgeries. He had stepped on a land mine, and they were doing skin grafts on his feet. He was in a wheelchair, and I was flat on my back, but he taught me to play cribbage. We played that game quite a bit to help pass the time.

It's hard for me to remember the exact ages and what they did when, but I think that when I was 10, they pinned the knee of my left leg, which is my "good" leg. That was done to slow down the growth. They wanted to do that procedure before I had my growth spurt so my legs wouldn't get too far out of balance.

About two years later, I had my third surgery. That one was a procedure called a "V-fistula." It was done to increase the rate of growth in my right leg. They did that by taking a vein and connecting it to an artery which increased the blood flow. That stimulated the growth. Because of that operation, the overall difference in the length of my legs is only about an eighth or a quarter of an inch, so I'd say it worked pretty well.

I believe the V-fistula was an experimental, or at least a new procedure at that time. I remember that I drew some pretty big crowds. All sorts of medical people from other countries would come into my room. They didn't speak English, at least not as their first language, and sometimes there'd be a couple of them in my room talking in whatever their language happened to be. At the time I thought that was pretty interesting.

A couple of years later, I had my fourth surgery. That one was performed to undo the V-fistula. They undid the procedure because it put an additional strain on my heart. I remember getting examined by heart specialists to make sure everything was okay. The vein where they did that surgery would sort of buzz when you touched the skin above it. If you listened with a stethoscope, you could really hear it, so I know the blood was rushing through there. I think it was the plan all along to undo it after I completed my growth spurt.

Even after all that, I still wasn't done with my surgeries. I had two more, the next one probably coming when I was about 15. During that surgery, I think they did some work on the bones of my right foot. They also tried to tighten the tendons to keep my big toe from dropping.

Unfortunately, the toe surgery didn't take. Someone stepped on my toe on the school bus shortly after I got out of the hospital. I'm not sure if that resulted in the problem or not, but my mom thinks that's what did it. Whatever the reason, the toe started dropping again, so the next summer I was back in the hospital for my sixth surgery. This time, they took a chip of bone from my right shin and fused it into the toe to hold it straight. The surgery worked, and the toe has stayed straight. However, the fused toe has caused me some problems. Since the toe won't bend, I tend to stub it a lot, and I've actually taken the skin off of it on a few occasions.

That toe surgery was done when I was 16. I haven't had any surgeries since then, which is very nice. However, even though the surgeries were successful, I still walk with a limp and was left with two different size legs and feet. I wear a size six shoe on one foot and a four and a half on the other, so I'm between women's and children's sizes. I used to just buy the larger size and stuff something in the toe. It was less noticeable that way. However, as I've gotten older and my feet have grown wider, I've been going to a special shoe store where they can order shoes in the two different sizes for me. It's more expensive, but the shoes are a lot more comfortable.

My asymmetrical feet and legs made adolescence difficult for me. I think adolescence is a difficult time for everyone, but when you have a visible difference, it makes it even harder. In a way, I was fortunate because I entered junior high school just about the time when you didn't have to wear dresses to school anymore. Being able to wear pants to school saved me a lot of embarrassment.

Other than being self-conscious about my legs, I think I got through high school pretty well. I didn't date, and I didn't go to school dances, and I'm sure that was probably because of polio, but otherwise, I did pretty much everything everyone else did. I was even in regular P.E. There were some things that I couldn't do, like track, but I was a strong swimmer, and I even played volleyball. I never felt like I was singled out because of something I couldn't do.

I was a good student in high school. In fact, I took extra classes so that I could graduate early and go to college. I went to the University of Minnesota for a while, and I also attended Metropolitan Community College, but I never got a degree. I ended up just having pieces of different degrees.

Even though I didn't finish a degree, I do have a very good career. I do computer work for U.S. West, and I make a pretty good income, which I need to do because since my husband and I got divorced, I've been pretty much supporting myself and my three children.

As far as my current situation, I think I'm doing quite well. I'm fortunate in that I haven't experienced any new weakness or excessive fatigue. However, I have been using a cane when I have to walk any distance. I started to use it when I was pregnant. It was suggested to me when I was 17 that I use a cane, but when you're a teenager, the last thing you want to do is walk with a cane. I do walk with a limp,

and occasionally someone will ask me about it. I don't mind that.
They just are curious and want to know.

I have a handicapped parking sticker; I first got a temporary one
in 1984 when I was pregnant. Then in 1985 I got a permanent one.
I don't use handicapped parking all the time, though. If there are a
lot of spots available, I'll use one, but if there's just one handicapped
spot open, I won't take it. There might be somebody else who needs
it more than I do.

I don't believe that I have post-polio syndrome. I have read quite
a bit about it, though. When the information about exercise first came
out, I started riding a stationary bike. I worked up to where I was
riding it for 20 minutes, four times a week, but then I got bronchitis
and hurt my back, so I slowed down a little. I also ride a regular bike
when the weather allows. My bike is sort of in between a children's
and adult's size because my legs are so short. Some days I feel like
I could ride forever, and it doesn't phase me at all. If I go up and
down a lot of hills though, then I'll get tired and need to rest, but I
do enjoy biking, especially with my kids.

Recently, I have had some unusual symptoms that I wonder about.
I get goose bumps on the right side of my body. Mostly I get them
on my right leg, from my thigh to my hip. Occasionally I get them
on my right arm. It's not that I'm cold; the goose bumps just appear
for no reason, and always on my right side. I can't help but wonder
if the goose bumps are in some way related to my polio. I'm thinking
of making an appointment to have a post-polio evaluation done at
Sister Kenny Institute. Like I said, I don't seem to have any serious
problems, but I'd like to get my situation evaluated and find out what
I can do to prevent problems from developing.

As far as whether anything good came from my having had polio,
I believe that my disability makes it easier for my kids to relate to
others who are handicapped. For instance, my middle daughter has
a girl in her class who wears hearing aids, and she really doesn't
think anything of it. All my kids seem to relate quickly and easily to
handicapped children.

It's hard for me to even imagine what my life might have been like
if I wouldn't have had polio. Thinking about a life with two normal
feet and legs and without all my surgeries doesn't seem real to me.
I know I would have been three inches taller, so I wouldn't have
always been the "short one." Maybe I would have dated in high
school. Perhaps I would have even been athletic, but who knows?
And when I was a child, my parents allowed me to do pretty much

anything I wanted, so I really don't feel like I was cheated out of a normal childhood. In fact, I had a good childhood, and I think I've had a pretty good adulthood as well.

Chapter 5

Scoliosis: The Abnormal Curve

Those whose polio affected their trunk muscles often developed scoliosis, or curvature of the spine. In some cases, the curvature was severe enough to require prolonged bracing, casting, or even spinal fusion surgery, an operation that straightened the spine by placing chips of bone between the vertebrae.

The three individuals whose stories appear in this chapter all had spinal fusion surgery as a result of their polio and subsequent scolioses. All three surgeries were successful. However, two of the three developed "complications" that resulted in additional surgeries.

It is interesting to note that the three of us whose stories appear in this chapter all had polio in 1953. That must have been a very good year for scolioses! Though scoliosis is the common feature in these three stories, there is much more to them. Therefore, they are presented in their entirety.

Edmund Sass

I don't remember a great deal about my early childhood years, but those memories I do have are very happy ones. We lived in a rural area, and I know that I loved to go across the road to visit my grandparents and try to catch the tadpoles, frogs, and turtles that lived in their pond. I also remember that my dad used to pitch me baseballs quite often, but I seldom hit them. I was too distracted by the birds and bugs and other creatures that inhabited our yard. I loved to go "exploring" in the fields and woods around our home, and I was always looking under rocks and logs to see what I might find there. My mom often had to come looking for me so that I wouldn't miss my lunch or supper. Unfortunately though, my childhood changed abruptly in early June of 1953. It was then that I came down with polio. I was six years old at the time.

My mom tells me that a family friend had come to our home and had brought along a three or four-year-old girl who was visiting them. Though I don't remember, apparently the little girl was very sick. My mom says that she was complaining about having a stiff neck and feeling very tired. Based on what I know now, I assume I caught polio from that little girl.

A few days later, my mom became very ill, probably with non-paralytic polio. She recalls having the classic symptoms: fever, nausea, headache, and a stiff neck. She must have really been sick, because my mom was over-protective, but the day before I came down with polio, she allowed me to play the whole day at a neighbor's house. I didn't even come home for lunch. She never would have allowed me to do that if she had been well.

Apparently I came home exhausted, which may have predisposed me to the major, paralytic form of polio. I started having symptoms that night. My parents tell me that I awakened them in the middle of the night complaining that I was having "attacks" in my legs. I guess I was experiencing pain and muscle spasms.

The next morning, my parents called our family doctor, and he came out and examined me. He must have suspected polio right away because he had my parents carry me around, even to and from the bathroom.

I didn't get any better, so later that day, the doctor had my parents take me to the hospital. I remember my dad carrying me into the hospital and getting the obligatory spinal tap, but I remember very little else about my stay in the hospital. I do know that I didn't get the Sister Kenny treatment that so many of the other individuals we interviewed received. I'm not sure why, but instead of wrapping my limbs in hot, moist compresses, I was given six shots a day, at least some of which were injections of curare. I looked it up. Curare is a poison that South American tribes used to dip their arrows in. It paralyzed the animals that were struck by the arrows.

Can you imagine that? They injected my already paralyzed muscles with a poison to paralyze them even further. I guess the theory was that the curare would stop the spasms and allow the muscles to be stretched and manipulated. I once asked a physician knowledgeable about polio treatments if the use of curare was effective. He just smiled and said, "Well, it gave them something to do." I wish they hadn't done it to me! My little rear end must have looked like a pin cushion. To this day I can't stand needles. When I get a shot or have blood drawn, I have to look the other way. I can't even stand to watch someone get a shot on T.V.

I was only in the hospital three or four weeks. Since virtually everyone else I interviewed was hospitalized for a much longer time, I recently asked my mother if she knew why my stay in the hospital was so relatively brief. She told me that it was because the Polio Foundation wouldn't cover my medical expenses, and we had reached the maximum amount that our insurance would cover. Apparently if we had lived in a different county, the expenses would have been covered, but not in Cook County, Illinois. They told my parents to take a second mortgage on their home. And it wasn't that we were wealthy. My dad was a carpenter, and as was the case with most women of that era, my mom was a homemaker with three young children.

My dad ended up having to work side jobs, at night and on the weekends, to pay the medical bills. I once asked him what the total cost of my polio-related expenses was. He really didn't know. I guess those sort of expenses aren't the kind of thing of which one keeps a running count. Rather, you just keep trying to pay them and hope you don't lose your home in the process.

So, obviously, my illness and all that was to follow must have been really difficult on my parents. But I have a younger brother and sister, and I've often wondered what the impact of all this was on them. We've never talked about it, but seeing all of our parents' energy and so much of the family's resources go to me must have been very difficult for them as well.

At any rate, when I was released from the hospital, they told my parents that I probably would never be able to walk again. Shortly after coming home, however, I got out of bed and walked to the bathroom. I fell down at the bathroom door. My mom came running over. She was crying and hugging me, and said, "You can walk!." Though I don't remember saying it, my mom tells me that I replied, "You didn't think I'd forgotten already; did you?." All my life I've been vain enough to think it was remarkable that I've not only been able to walk, but to walk without crutches or canes. However, since I've been doing this project, I've found that many of the people I interviewed were told that they'd never walk again; and virtually all of them walk, or at least used to be able to walk. So I guess my being able to walk is not particularly remarkable after all.

I started school that fall. We had a two-room school. First through fourth grades were in one room and fifth through eighth in the other. They had just built the new two-room addition that year. The old one-room schoolhouse was closed up and just used for storage.

I don't have great memories about my elementary school days. In a small school like that, of course, everyone knew I had polio, and for the most part, they treated me very well. There was no teasing, at least not during first grade, and the children included me in their games. However, I was never very good at the games, particularly if they involved running. I was always the slowest runner in the entire school, and sometimes the kids would avoid choosing me for their teams. Not that I blame them, but my poor running ability caused me much pain and embarrassment. When I complained to my mother about my inability to run well, she just said, "Well, you had polio." I couldn't argue with her, and unfortunately, that answer was to explain many other aspects of my life.

I know I had some physical therapy for a year or two after I got out of the hospital. I remember going either to a clinic or hospital and getting stretched and twisted in all sorts of painful directions. I also remember getting "electrical stimulation" to see if my stomach muscles could somehow be jump-started. It didn't work, of course.

I did some stretching and strengthening exercises at home. The exercise I remember the best involved grasping a five pound lead weight as I lay on the floor and kind of heaving it over my head to give me enough momentum to do a sit-up. To this day that's still the only way I can do one.

There was also some sort of swimming program. I believe that we used a private, indoor pool in Wilmette (a ritzy Chicago suburb). The family that owned the pool donated its use. Perhaps one of their children was a polio victim. Though I must have gone there many times, I only really remember one of them. My mom didn't drive at that time, so other women who belonged to our church would take turns driving me. On this particular occasion, Mrs. Widerow (who was also my piano teacher) took me. We must have been almost there when one of us noticed that I didn't have my swimming suit. Well, Mrs. Widerow gave me this lecture that went something like, "Are you going to be a brave boy and swim in your underwear, or are you going to be a spineless coward and refuse to swim." What could I say? I swam in my underwear. I don't think I was embarrassed about it, but I can only imagine what the other people thought. It's funny the incidents that stick in your memory.

Believe it or not, I was given the Salk vaccine during the second grade. I believe it was in the spring, probably May, 1955. Therefore, I must have been among the very first to have been vaccinated. I remember that they loaded up the whole school and took us to the neighboring town of Glenview, where we all lined up to get the vaccine. I told the doctor or whoever was giving the injections that I didn't need the vaccine because I had already had polio. He just smiled and stuck the needle in my arm. Perhaps he wanted to make sure I didn't get it again!

I must have started developing a scoliosis about that same time. I remember being x-rayed in my family doctor's office, probably starting some time during second grade. The x-rays were apparently sent to an orthopedic doctor in Chicago who monitored my scoliosis. He thought my family physician was taking the x-rays of me in a standing position, whereas he was actually taking them with me lying down. Therefore, the orthopedic doctor didn't think the scoliosis was as bad as it really was until I saw him in person. Basically, he said our family doctor was an idiot and that I needed to be immediately fitted with a Milwaukee brace.

If you've never seen a Milwaukee brace, it's quite a contraption. The bottom is made of leather which fits around your hips and pelvis and buckles up in front. I wore that part under my pants. There is a long metal bar that attaches to the leather and runs up the front. That goes outside of your clothes. It extends up to your neck where it attaches to a padded chin rest. The chin rest bolts to an additional padded piece that fits behind your neck. And, of course, another bar attaches to that and extends down your back where it connects to the bottom leather. Mine also had a leather strap that fit around my side to hold in my scoliosis. I guess it was the ultimate portable traction device. I wore that thing nearly 24 hours a day.

I vividly remember the first day that I wore the brace to school. It was the middle of the school day. Apparently, I had gone to the doctor that morning to have the brace fitted. My mom dropped me off at the door, and as I approached the room, I heard somebody say, "Here he comes!" I guess they were expecting me. After I took my seat, the teacher asked me if I wanted to say anything to the class. Everyone was staring at me with great anticipation. I think I managed a feeble, "No." I just wanted to hide under the desk.

For days, maybe weeks thereafter, that Milwaukee brace was the major topic of conversation around the school. It was almost like the other children were delighted to have this new curiosity in their midst. Eventually, of course, the novelty wore off, and things basically returned to normal.

Outside of school though, nobody knew what a Milwaukee brace was or why I was wearing it, so I used to get a lot of stares and questions. When I'd tell other kids that I wore the brace because I had polio, they'd often say something like, "Boy, are you lucky." I could never really understand that reaction. I guess they meant I was "lucky" that I wasn't dead or in an iron lung. However, it always seemed to me that if I had really been lucky, I never would have gotten the damned disease in the first place.

I got so tired of explaining why I wore the brace that when other kids would ask me about it, I'd say, "Well, my dad's a carpenter, and one day he got careless with the electric saw and cut my head off. The brace holds it on." The looks I got were amazing. What's even more amazing is how many kids believed that's really why I wore the brace!

I think it was the summer after third grade that I spent a week in Williams Bay, Wisconsin with my grandparents. It was probably a treat to try and take my mind off of the brace. Every day I was there, we would walk the couple of blocks to Lake Geneva, and I would fish off of the dock. I remember that I met this little blond girl from Milwaukee who was staying there for the summer. She would also come down to the dock, and we would fish together. I really liked that little girl, not because I had a crush on her, but because during that whole week, she never once asked me about the brace. Somehow, I got it in my head that since she was from Milwaukee, she must know all about Milwaukee braces. Probably, she was just too polite to ask.

I wore the brace or some variant of it for about the next five years. I played baseball in it, played football, and did, or at least tried, all the typical things that boys do. I did get to take the brace off for Little League baseball games. I wasn't much of a fielder. I had pretty good coordination and could catch the ball well, but I couldn't run very far to get it. So I ended up playing first base. I was a pretty good batter, but I had bad reflexes and had a lot of trouble getting out of the way of inside pitches. Therefore, I got hit by pitches quite often. That fact as well as the pressure of the games always made me very nervous, and I didn't enjoy Little League, but at least I got to take the brace off when I played.

About the only other time I got to take the brace off was if it got wet. I remember one incident when it got so wet that I couldn't wear it for two or three days. I had stayed overnight at my friend Carter's house, and we decided to make a boat, so we took one of his father's wheelbarrows and unbolted the frame and handles. Carter's dad was a chemist, and we used some of his test tube stoppers to plug up the holes where the bolts had gone. We carried that "boat" to a large pond and got in. We hadn't gotten very far before our makeshift boat sank. Fortunately, we could both swim, or we would have gone down with the ship. The water was so deep, however, that we couldn't get the wheelbarrow out. Carter's mom was a good sport and thought the whole incident was funny, though I'm sure his dad didn't feel that way. Neither did my mom. I'll never forget the look on her face when she came to pick me up and saw that soaking-wet brace hanging on the clothes line. I did enjoy the next couple of days without wearing it though.

One incident related to the brace that has more or less haunted me occurred when I was about 10 years old. I was on a shopping trip with my mother, and as we were entering a store, we were confronted by a little man who was begging or selling pencils or something. He had the worst scoliosis I've ever seen. His back was incredibly twisted and deformed, and his shoulders were almost down to his hips. He saw my brace and asked my mom why I was wearing it. She told him that I had polio and was wearing the brace because I had developed a curvature of the spine. The man laughed and said something like, "Well, that's what I had. He's going to end up just like me." My mom told him that I was wearing the brace so I wouldn't end up like him. He laughed what I recall as being a particularly sinister sort of laugh and just kept repeating, "We'll see. We'll see," as we walked into the store.

We left by a different exit, and I never saw that man again. However, I thought about him for weeks or maybe even months thereafter. I even had nightmares about him. Though that event happened nearly 40 years ago, I can still vividly picture him standing there laughing. I've often wondered what became of him, but perhaps it's better that I don't know.

The only time the brace ever came in handy was during eighth grade when I was involved in a fight. I remember that I walked into the boys' bathroom and saw a boy named Ralph sticking my classmate Arthur's head in the urinal. I didn't know what the fight was about, but Arthur had cerebral palsy, and was no match for

Ralph. When I tried to intervene, Ralph hit me in the head. Though I didn't know it at the time, Ralph had broken his hand when he punched me. With him partially disabled, I was able to get his head sort of caught up inside the front of my brace. I held onto the brace with both hands, and even though he squealed and squirmed with all his might, Ralph couldn't escape. For the next few seconds, Arthur proceeded to kick and punch Ralph as hard and as often as a guy with spasticity possibly could. Fortunately for us all, the fight was quickly broken up.

Though I remember the principal being quite angry with us, I don't believe we really received any punishment. The next day, however, Ralph came to school with a cast on his hand, and his dad was overheard yelling at the principal and wanting to know how she could have allowed a couple of cripples to beat up his son!

A few days later we had a spring snowstorm. Arthur and I wanted to shoot baskets, so we spent most of our lunch hour shoveling off the outdoor basketball court. As we walked back to our classroom, we passed Ralph. Arthur looked at him and said, "Hey Ralph, if your dad wants to know who shoveled off the basketball court, just tell him it was a couple of cripples!" Ralph just smiled. He really wasn't such a bad guy. I think he just had a lot of problems at home. Actually, the three of us got along quite well the rest of that spring. Ralph even let Arthur and me sign his cast.

Some time during that spring, my orthopedic doctor died. I was referred to a physician named Immerman who took over my case. He was quite a character. Though he was nice to me, he used to rant and rave at the nurses. Sometimes he would swear at them in Polish. I didn't understand what he was saying, but my dad speaks Polish fluently. He would often smile and roll his eyes during these outbursts.

After he saw me for the first time, Dr. Immerman told my parents that my previous treatment had been all wrong and that I needed a body cast. So, that's what I got! I remember my dad took me down to a hospital in Chicago, and they hung me on this contraption, covered me with a body sock, and wrapped me in plaster from my hips to my arm pits. I can vividly recall the smell and feel of that warm plaster. I believe the process of molding that cast took about three hours. I wasn't allowed to move, and I recall the event as being painful and terrifying. For years, I had dreams, or I should say nightmares, about that day and that cast.

I went home in the cast and basically wore it or a replacement for about the next two and one-half years. Of course, I couldn't take it off, and I believe it was changed only about every three months. Therefore, I could only take sponge baths. It was heavy, pinched the nerves in my hips, and sometimes I'd itch terribly. When that was the case, I'd take the vacuum cleaner and put on the attachment for getting down between tight places. I'd reverse the flow of the air and stick it down the cast. It felt great!

I started high school that fall, and it was a difficult time for me. I moved from my small elementary school, with a graduating class of 13 and where I knew everybody, to a high school with over 2000 students. I rarely saw a familiar face. For the most part, the other students weren't overtly cruel to me. Rather, they just avoided me. I can't say that I blame them. Wearing that bulky body cast, I must have looked awful and smelled worse.

I found the school day exhausting. I caught the bus at about 7:00 A.M. and got home about 4:00 P.M. The cast had to weigh at least 20 pounds, and lugging it around all day was about all I could handle. I did poorly in school that year; I got mostly C's. I'm sure that just surviving took most of my energy, and I had very little left over for my studies.

I had "modified P.E." my freshman year. There were boys with all sorts of physical limitations in that class. A few were recovering from surgery, but most had some permanent disability like cerebral palsy or a birth defect. We spent most of our time in the weight room, though I recall that we did play ping-pong and badminton. The other kids, of course, teased us about being in "spastic P.E.," but the teacher treated us well, and we developed sort of a comradery. So being in "spastic P.E." wasn't all that bad.

One would think that in such a large high school there would have been many other students who had polio, and maybe there were. However, to the best of my knowledge there was only one other person in that school who had any noticeable polio-related disability. His one leg was atrophied, and I remember hearing that he had a surgery to stop the growth in his "good" leg. Of course, we each knew that the other had had polio, but we never talked about it. I guess neither of us was quite ready for a support group right then.

The summer after my freshman year, I had my first back surgery. Dr. Immerman and Dr. Fisher, who I believe came to Chicago from Canada to do my surgery, did a spinal fusion to straighten up my scoliosis as much as was possible. The procedure involved putting little chips of bone between the vertebrae which eventually would grow together and form one solid, fused spinal column. Fortunately, the chips of bone that they inserted came from the "bone bank." Most people I've talked to who had similar surgeries had pieces of bone chipped from their hip.

The fusion was held in place by a long piece of steel called a Harrington rod which was attached to the top and bottom of the spine where the fusion ended. The insertion of the "rod" was a very new procedure at that time. In the six or seven hours that it took to do the surgery, my spine was straightened to the extent that I went from being about 5'6" to 6' tall. My spine still isn't completely straight, though. I would probably be about 6'4" if not for what's left of my scoliosis.

I think I was in the hospital for about three weeks. One incident that I clearly recall occurred shortly after the surgery. They removed me from my room and wheeled me down to this auditorium in which a bunch of what I assume were medical and nursing students were seated. Dr. Fisher then explained my surgery to the students as he changed my dressings. Lying there naked on that table while a physician talked about me like I was a scientific exhibit was a humiliating experience for a 14-year-old to have to endure. Fortunately, at least the incision was in my back, so I was lying on my side looking away from the audience.

Before I went home, they fit me with another full body cast to hold me upright and protect the fusion while it was healing. I was still wearing it when I started school in the fall. As far as I remember, that cast was about the same as the one I had worn the year before. It extended from my hips to my arm pits, was heavy, and very uncomfortable. The start of the school year was again exhausting, but by spring I was feeling well enough to shoot some baskets in the gym. I guess I shouldn't have done that. I felt a stabbing pain in the top of my back. When I reached under the cast, I felt quite a lump. The Harrington rod had come unhooked and was trying to poke itself out of my back. Needless to say, I was back in surgery shortly thereafter to have it removed. The doctors didn't seem to think the removal of the rod was such a big deal. They told my parents that about half of them eventually had to be taken out. I guess orthopedic medicine wasn't a very exact science. It probably still isn't.

Not too long after the removal of the rod, I had the last cast cut off. It was the best day of my young life. Of course, up to that point, I hadn't had that many other good days!

They then fit me with a fiberglass jacket. It was about the same dimensions as the body cast, but much thinner and lighter. Most importantly, I could take it off to shower. I felt like I was in heaven.

Some time during my junior year of high school, I was given the go ahead to dump the fiberglass jacket. After about eight years, I was finally brace, cast, and jacket-free. I could actually feel my skin against the sheets at night. I could walk and sit and even run a little without pain. I remember that whenever I had felt really down about my braces, casts, and other problems, my dad would always tell me something like, "You've got some really good years ahead. The best is yet to come." Well, it finally came. I felt like a normal person for the first time that I could recall.

During my senior year of high school, my polio was only occasionally a limiting factor and a cause of minor embarrassment, and it seemed like my life had improved infinitely. I couldn't participate in any sports, or I should say that I wasn't good enough to participate in any interscholastic sports in high school, and I didn't have a girlfriend, but otherwise, I did almost all the typical things that a high school student does. I even played on intramural football and basketball teams. I think our flag-football team lost every game, and my basketball team won only one game, but that really wasn't important. I got to do some of the things that were appropriate for kids my age for the first time in several years.

I actually even took regular P.E. during my senior year. My asymmetrical body made me embarrassed and self-conscious when I had swimming in gym class or when I was in the shower room, and there were also some things that I just couldn't do in gym class. I remember that we had to do all of the "president's physical fitness tests" in gym. We'd all line up and do the test and then get in another line to report our score. Well, when we were supposed to do one that I couldn't do, like number of sit-ups in a minute (my score would have been zero), I would simply wait a while and then get in the line to report the score. I'd listen to what the other scores were, and then just report one that was respectable, but a little below average. If the coach knew what I was doing, he was nice enough never to confront me about it. Actually, I think my P.E. teacher was quite sensitive to my situation. For instance, I remember that when we played basketball in gym, my team always kept our shirts on. The other team was always the "skins." I'm sure he knew that playing basketball in the gym without my t-shirt would have been embarrassing for me. I wish now that I would have thanked him for his kindness.

I went to college the next fall, and though I was certainly not a "big man on campus" I spent a relatively normal four years as an undergraduate. I ended up majoring in psychology, largely because I couldn't figure out anything else in which to major. With that major and essentially no skills, I had trouble finding a job and eventually went to work selling advertising for the *Chicago Tribune*. Sitting all day in the car as I drove around calling on accounts was hard on my back, but I was relatively successful. No one with whom I worked knew that I'd had polio, but now and then someone would notice my limp and ask if I had sprained my ankle. I never knew exactly how to answer them. I think that many people with disabilities that are not obvious must have similar predicaments. It's difficult to know whether to take the time to explain your situation to other people.

My boss at the *Tribune* eventually noticed my scoliosis and called me into his office. He told me that I had poor posture which might make a bad impression with some of my accounts. He suggested that perhaps I should consult a doctor or a physical therapist to see if my posture could be improved. When I explained that I had a scoliosis and a spinal fusion due to polio, his jaw just dropped. He never mentioned my posture again, and perhaps it was my imagination, but I thought that he never regarded me very highly after that. It really didn't matter. I never intended to make sales my life's work, and after about two years at the *Tribune*, I quit to go to graduate school.

It was during graduate school that I discovered I was a very good student. Though I had always done well on standardized tests, my grades in high school and college had only been a little above average. As a graduate student, however, I was really interested in my course work, and to my surprise, I started to do very well. I often got the highest scores on exams and received many compliments from teachers and my fellow students. I think that was the first time in my life I actually felt I was good at something.

I also learned another thing about myself during graduate school. In a counseling class that I was taking, we had to role-play counseling clients as other class members practiced using the various counseling techniques we were learning. The sessions were taped; the class would listen to the tapes, and we would critique each other. When we listened to the tapes on which I had role-played a client, my classmates often commented that I was a difficult person with whom to work because I did not express my feelings. Rather, I tended to intellectualize everything. When I thought about it, I could see why. I probably became very adept at denying or at least repressing my feelings as a child. I believe that if I had dealt with how I felt during the eight years I was wearing the braces and body casts, I would have been hysterical 24 hours a day. So not dealing with my feelings was probably a necessity for me. I have gotten better at expressing feelings over the years, but it hasn't been an easy process.

Between my studies, I started going to the gym and working out with the weight machines. I also played basketball and started playing tennis. I got really physically fit, I think for the first time in my life, and I was actually a pretty decent tennis player. Not that I could compete with advanced-level players, but I was a very good intermediate-level player. I still play at least twice a week, and doctors have told me that playing tennis is probably one major reason why I've been able to function as well as I have for these last 20 years.

After graduate school, I worked as a school psychologist for several years before more graduate studies and another career change brought me to college teaching. I've been at my present job at the College of Saint Benedict here in Minnesota since 1977. I am currently Director of Teacher Education, and I enjoy my work very much. I am married and have a terrific wife and three wonderful children. So I've had 30 very good years since that last cast was removed. Of course, I'd rather not have my scoliosis and my other polio-related problems. Who wouldn't want a normal, healthy body? But I've been like this for so long, and I'm really quite satisfied with my life.

I would like to be able to say with confidence that I know my life will continue basically as it is, and that I will be able to work and be physically active until I reach a normal retirement age. However, I don't know if that is realistic. From what I have seen and read, I know that many of us experience new or more pronounced polio-related problems as we age, and so I worry about the future.

Some days when I have more than my usual number of aches and pains or when my energy level is particularly low, I feel like I have a ticking time-bomb inside my body that is about to go off. I've come to the conclusion that polio is a particularly cruel disease. It steals your childhood, gives you 20 or 30 years to adjust to the disabilities with which you were left, and then threatens to return to complicate your life once again.

Apparently, that's what has been happening to me. Over these last two or three years, I have been experiencing some symptoms that concern me. I have had increasing back pain as well as new aches and pains in my neck and legs.

I've made several recent trips down to Sister Kenny Institute to have my situation evaluated and have been very impressed with the physicians there. During each visit, I spent about an hour talking with and being examined by the doctors. They listened; they cared; they understood; and most importantly, they had some ideas regarding how to help me.

They tell me that my leg and arm strength is still normal, and my cardio-vascular endurance is actually above average for a person my age. My aches and pains appear to be due to my scoliosis and/or are manifestations of the "unexplained joint and muscle pain" that go along with polio's late effects. However, I don't seem to be experiencing the progressive loss of strength that so many other polio survivors are reporting. Therefore, for now at least, my problems should be manageable with exercise, stretching, and knowing my limitations as far as what I should and shouldn't do.

I know that I'll continue to have at least my share of aches and pains. I've started to wear an upper back support when I do yard work or other strenuous activities. I'm also taking a medication to improve my energy level. But my job is not physically demanding, and I'm optimistic that I'll be able to continue working at least until I'm well into my 50's.

I exercise daily. I'm not sure if it helps, but I generally feel better after exercising, and, if nothing else, it helps me feel like I'm doing something to improve or at least maintain my current physical status. I know this sounds strange, but I actually feel best when I'm out playing tennis, mowing the lawn, or working in the garden.

I know that not everyone doing research on the late effects of polio agrees that exercise is beneficial. I've read about the group in California that recommends "babying your motor neurons" and "listening to your body." But if I listened to mine, I'm afraid that all I'd do is sit on the couch and complain, and I'm sure not ready to do that. Instead, I intend to keep exercising and living my life basically as I have. I also intend to see a physician at Sister Kenny Institute at least once a year for my own peace of mind and to make sure that I'm doing the right things. I have a very good life, and I intend to do everything I can to keep it that way for as long as possible.

Carole Sauer

I was 10 years old in 1953. That year marks an important point in my life, because it was during the summer of 1953 that I was diagnosed with polio.

The day that the symptoms began, I was out mowing the lawn, and I remember that I was not feeling well at all. My whole body just ached. My mom and dad called our doctor, and he thought I should go into the hospital, but I really didn't want to go. However, my mom and dad decided to follow the doctor's advice, so some time that evening, they took me in. We had a pickup truck, and we had to go down a bumpy road. It seemed like such a long ride. Every time we hit a bump, I just hurt all over.

I was admitted to St. Cloud Hospital that night, and I went right into the isolation ward. If I remember correctly, that ward was down in the basement. That way, they could keep all the polio patients separated from everyone else. My bed was next to that of about a three-year-old child, and in the next bed over, there was a girl about my age.

I remember being scared to death. They really didn't tell you what was going on, and back in those days, you didn't dare ask, but I have a vivid memory of them pushing my bed out in the hall right next to this iron lung machine. I still remember the noise the machine made. It gave me such an eery feeling. I thought that I was going to be put into that iron lung. Fortunately, I never was put in it, but just being out there next to that machine was a very frightening experience. Probably the scariest thing about that isolation ward though, was the separation from my parents. We were allowed no visitors at all.

Eventually, I started to get the treatment with the hot packs. The treatment was just like the advertisement from that era for St. Cloud Hospital. They would heat up these blankets in an old wringer washing machine; they'd run them through the wringer, and then they'd wrap us up in them. They covered up my whole body with those things.

I think they did that treatment with us three or four times a day. Being covered with the hot blanket helped to reduce the achiness a lot. I got to the point were after three or four hours, I could only feel the heat, not the pain.

There's one incident I remember from my stay in the hospital that I think is kind of interesting. One day an intern came around and told me, "We're going to take some blood from you. I know that you have polio, so we're going to be using your blood to make a serum." After he took the blood, he said, "Just think of the hundreds of people you're going to be helping." I didn't really understand it at the time, but apparently they took my blood to help make the polio vaccine.

A couple of years later, I actually got vaccinated against polio. I remember that after the vaccine came out, we asked the doctor if I needed it. He said, "Yes, you definitely need it, because there is more than one type of polio." So, even though I already had polio, I still had to keep up with my vaccinations.

Anyway, I'm really not sure how long I was in the hospital. It may have been only about 10 days or two weeks. They released me relatively quickly because of how crowded the hospital was, and I guess they needed my bed. Since I was recovering pretty well, they thought I could continue my treatment at home. Also, I was an only child, and the doctor knew that. So he thought my mother would have the time to take care of me.

By the time I got out of the hospital, I was able to walk, at least a little. I was still very weak, however, and my mom continued the treatment with the hot packs for quite a while. She got an old blanket, heated it up in her washing machine, ran it through the wringer, and then would wrap me in it. I'd say she did that for two months or so. Then she had to do therapy with me. I remember that she had me do exercises with my legs and arms. We also did exercises with my neck because I was unable to lift up my head.

Within a few months, I had recovered pretty well, but I started to develop a curvature of the spine. I remember that my mom would always be telling me to stand up straight, and I though that I was. She would take my shoulders and try to pull them straight, and then she'd say, "There, now you're straight. That's the way you should be." But it didn't feel right to me when she'd do that. I'd feel pulling in the spine, so that's when we went back to the doctor. I remember him saying he had kind of suspected that I'd get a curvature of the spine because the polio had hit my back more than any other part of my body. He referred us to a specialist in St. Paul, and when I was 12, which was two years after my initial bout with polio, I was back in the hospital for surgery on my spine. This time I was in for a rather lengthy stay.

I actually had two spinal surgeries, one right after the other. My curvature of the spine was pretty severe and had started to form an "S" shape, so it took two surgeries to straighten it out. During the surgeries, they put little chips of bone along side my spine. Actually, I was quite lucky in that they didn't have to chip bones from other parts of my body to use in the surgeries. I understand that the surgery to chip the bone out was even more painful than the back surgery. But fortunately, the doctor told us that they had a "bone bank." It was a new experiment, sort of like a "blood bank." They used bone from that "bone bank" for my operations, so apparently I have pieces of bone from someone else in my back.

Back in those days, they were still using ether for general anesthesia. They would put a mask over your face and drop ether on the mask. Well, they missed the mask with one drop, and got it in my eye. It burned terribly, and I couldn't see out of that eye for at least a week. They thought I might lose the sight in that eye, but I recovered my sight completely.

After my surgeries, they put me in a full body cast. It extended from my neck down almost to my knees. Having it put on was quite an ordeal. It took several hours, and I had to lie on these straps, just sort of balancing there, while they wrapped me in the plaster. The smell and feel of that warm plaster was sickening.

Having the cast put on once would have been bad enough, but I actually had to have it put on twice. Apparently, they should have stretched me out when they put the cast on, but they didn't. So, three days later, I had to go through the whole ordeal again. To make matters worse, when they cut off the first cast, they cut me with the saw. I guess you could say that wasn't a very good day for me!

I was in the hospital for a total of about two months, and I spent the whole year flat on my back in that full body cast. I couldn't get around at all, not even to get up and go to the bathroom. I had to use bed pans, which was pretty humiliating.

My dad worked with the St. Cloud Hospital, and he made this "cart" with wheelchair wheels in the front, and regular little wheels in the back. I would lie on that cart, and my parents could push me around in it. That way, at least I could get from one room to another. I remember that mom and dad would put these boards at both ends, and then they'd push it alongside the bed, and I could sort of scoot over onto it. That was the only way I could get out of bed for that entire year.

The cast was terribly uncomfortable, and I developed sores all around the edges where it rubbed against my skin. I itched terribly under the cast, and the only way I could relieve the itching was to take the end of a fly swatter and stick it in this little hole in the cast at the top of my neck. I'd try to reach down with the handle of that fly swatter and scratch as best I could.

I remember the day when I finally got that full body cast off. My skin was all red and scaly and just peeled off along with the cast. There was this little hole in the front of the cast where you could see my tummy, and my skin was a different color where that hole had been. It looked kind of like a tan line. Anyway, after I got that cast off, they just washed me off and put another cast on me which I had to wear for about another six months. The new cast was, more or less, a partial cast. This one didn't extend up as high in the back as my previous cast, and it allowed me to bend my legs a little, so I could start walking again.

I sure didn't start walking that very day though! Instead, I basically had to learn to walk all over again. I remember that right after they put the new cast on me, they sat me up, and it seemed like the room just started spinning around. I was so dizzy that I had to lie back down. I guess it took a while to have the blood go back to my head again or something. I was also very weak. After all, it had been a whole year since I had been on my feet. But it only took me a week or so before I was able to walk again, so it wasn't that bad. I do know that I was a little fearful of bending over for quite a while. I guess that I was afraid of breaking something.

I had a pretty positive attitude throughout this whole time period, and I think that helped a lot. I only remember one time that I really got down. My folks had company, and they had taken me outside on the cart my dad had made for me. They wheeled me down this plank that they had at the back door, and then when the company arrived, everyone just kind of forgot about me. I couldn't move, of course, and I felt completely neglected. I started crying and said, "Nobody loves me anymore!" That was about the only time I remember when I really felt down.

Other than that one incident, I really have to thank my mom and dad for all the things they did for me. For instance, I belonged to 4-H, and if the weather was nice, they'd load me up in the back of the pickup truck and haul me over for the 4-H meeting. I'd lie on the floor or the couch, and that way, I still got to see some of my friends.

I guess I did sort of think of myself as a burden on my family though, at least during the time I was in the full body cast. I think I held them down a lot. I couldn't do much for myself, and mom and dad had to do almost everything for me. I had baby sat for children before my surgery, but now with the cast on, I was so helpless that I needed a babysitter!

I was so happy when I was just able to get from one room to another and maybe get a book off of a shelf by myself and didn't have to bother my parents to do it for me. I'm sure they didn't mind, but never the less, I felt badly about having to ask them to do so many things for me.

My parents tell me that I never really felt sorry for myself, or at least, I never really acted like I did. However, I do remember that it bothered me when I'd see my friends outside playing ball or doing other things like that. My friends would come over to the house, and we'd play cards or board games, but I really missed being able to go out and play. I loved skating and playing sports, so being laid up for a whole year was very difficult.

At least I didn't get held back at all in school. I went to a little country school, and the teacher came over to my house every day after school to give me my lessons. That way I could keep up with all my school work.

After that partial cast was cut off, I was able to go back to school and return to a normal life again. I did have to go back to get checkups on my back until I was 21 years old, however. I remember the doctor telling me that I would have to be careful with my back because it would always be weak. I took his advice, and I have always been careful to watch my movement, especially bending. I can't do sit-ups, and I remember when I was in high school, I had to get a letter from the doctor so that I could be excused from doing hard, physical exercise.

Other than those limitations, I've lived a very normal life. I'm married and have three children. Most people that I meet don't even know that I had polio. They really can't tell by looking at me. Several times at work, we'd get to talking about polio, and I would say, "I'm one of the people who had it." The others would be really surprised because I look so healthy. Even if people see the scar on my back, they usually don't guess that it's from polio. My scar shows a little if I wear a certain type of top, and people will notice that and say, "What did you do to your back." When I tell them that I had polio and a spinal fusion, they're very surprised. So, I don't have a disability that is very noticeable to other people.

I know that I've been very fortunate to have gotten along as well as I have over the years, but lately I'm beginning to wonder if I'm starting to get some of those post-polio symptoms that I've read about. My hip that has always been a little weak has been bothering me more and more. I'm also getting neck pain. I wonder if it's from old age, arthritis, polio, or some combination.

I feel tired a lot, and sometimes I have shortness of breath. I guess I've had that for four or five years now. The other night, for instance, I was getting ready to go for a walk, and I was just so short of breath that I thought, "My gosh, how am I going to be able to walk if I can hardly breathe." But it's interesting. I feel better when I get out and exercise. I start taking a few deep breaths, and I feel okay again. I still go deer hunting, and I still enjoy working in my garden, though I am thinking that I'll plant my garden rows a little farther apart this year!

So I'm still doing pretty well in spite of having had polio, but I have, of course, thought about what things would be like if I hadn't had the disease. I'm sure my life would have been different, but I don't know if it would have been that much different. I guess I just think that if I hadn't gotten polio, I would have had a lot more fun. That probably would have been the major difference.

Sharon Kimball

About the first week of August, 1953, I spent a week at church camp. I had a complete physical before going to camp, and I was perfectly healthy, at least as far as we knew. I left for camp on a Monday morning and spent the week swimming, going on nature walks, and doing all the other things kids do at a summer camp. There was a lot to do, and I probably didn't get as much sleep as usual.

I got back to St. Cloud on Saturday, and that's when I began having symptoms. I remember feeling this strange sensation. It's hard to describe, but it was as though my head was under water. There was a ringing in my ears. I had a severe headache, and my vision was blurred. On Sunday, I felt very fatigued. I always sat with my mother in church, but that day, I was so tired that I had to lie down and put my head on her lap. My mom probably thought I was pouting or didn't want to be in church, but that wasn't the case. I just was feeling very ill.

I remember wanting so much to be well because I was back with my neighborhood friends whom I had missed when I was at camp. I wanted to play with them and tell them about my camp experiences. My girlfriend's rabbit had just had bunnies, but I was so tired that I almost had to drag myself over there to see them.

By Monday, my parents were becoming very concerned, and that evening, they called the doctor. He came out to our house on Tuesday morning and observed some of my symptoms. After taking my temperature, he told my parents that I needed to go to the hospital for a spinal tap.

After the spinal tap was done and the diagnosis of polio was made, I was immediately placed in isolation and told that I shouldn't raise my head. I remember that they put me in a crib! I was nine years old, and I couldn't understand why I had been placed in a crib. It was very degrading. I certainly wasn't going to climb out of bed, nor was I likely to roll over and fall out. In fact, I could hardly move. As I lay there in that crib, I could feel the virus really setting in. It was like a door slamming shut. I felt like my world had totally changed. To make things worse, it was terribly hot and humid, and of course, that was before air conditioning; I remember feeling very uncomfortable.

I spent about 10 days in isolation, and I couldn't have visitors, so I was again separated from my mother. I had just come through my first trip away from home, and now I was in isolation and away from the comfort of my family once again. My only connection to home was the telephone. I could call home, and my mom could call me. Dad talked too, but he didn't enjoy talking on the phone.

After a few days, they began whatever form of treatment was in vogue back then. I remember that we had to take some vile kinds of red and green liquids. I'm not sure if I had to take one or both, but I know that when the tray came around, I didn't want to drink either of them. My most vivid memory, however, is hearing the large, wringer washers being rolled down the hall. They used those washing machines to heat up the water in which they would dip green army blankets. Then they'd put them through the wringers and wrap our bodies in them. I believe they did that twice a day, maybe at 10 or 11 in the morning and then at about four or five in the afternoon. I was never one to be bothered by the heat, but the combination of the sultry August weather and those hot, moist blankets was very uncomfortable.

We also got hot baths, and I remember that there was a canvas in the tub which made sort of a hammock. They slid us onto that, and it was very comfortable. It felt warm and refreshing, and I sure enjoyed those baths a lot more than I did the army blankets, which were the other hot things in my life.

After isolation, I was moved up to the fourth floor where I was in a room that had five beds in it. I believe that there were over 300 people with polio in the St. Cloud Hospital that summer, so there was no such thing as a private or even a double room. Even the halls were filled with polio patients. I developed a close relationship with the girl who was in the bed next to me. I even visited her after I was out of the hospital. She was seven, and I was nine, but age really didn't matter when you had polio. We were both going through the same ordeal.

Another thing from my stay in the hospital that I particularly remember is that they brought us trays filled with too much food. I was a very small girl, and they would bring me a tray that went on forever, and they wanted me to eat it all. In fact, they would bribe, cajole, cheer, and do just about anything to get us to eat. I was a "people pleaser" by nature, so I ate as much of it as I possibly could. After about four weeks, the doctor looked at me and said I had put on a lot of weight, and he wondered if that extra weight would make it more difficult for me to get up and walk. I had been scarfing down all this food that I didn't even want just to please the people around me, and then they were worried that I had put on too much weight. It would seem to me that it wouldn't have taken a rocket scientist to figure out that someone should have been watching my diet all along!

When I was well enough, they began a physical therapy program. I remember doing a lot of leg lifts and stretches to keep my hamstring muscles from tightening up. My legs were initially almost completely paralyzed, so at first, I couldn't even lift them up off of the bed. And I had been a very active child up to that point. I was a runner and a jumper, and I was always hanging from the jungle gyms. So I felt pretty demoralized by the extent of my paralysis. However, one day while I was getting a hot bath, my therapist told me to try some leg lifts. When your legs are under water, of course, it's much easier to lift them, and I was able to lift them a little. I remember that sensation of actually being able to move my legs again. It was glorious! I guess if you've never been paralyzed, being able to move your legs a little doesn't seem like much of an accomplishment, but believe me; it was, and we were all pretty excited about it.

Something else that really sticks in my mind is the time I spent out on the sun porch. I remember going out to that sun porch very well. It was a pretty big event because it sort of marked a re-entry into life for me. The nurses took us out there in our wheelchairs, and the sun in our faces and the wind in our hair was glorious. I remember being out on that porch one day and smelling the tar, the wonderful hot, black tar that was such a familiar summer smell back then. To me, the smell of that tar was the essence of my childhood summers because we would go wherever they were putting tar on the neighborhood roads and watch the machines work. So the smell of the tar made me feel like there was some hope of getting back to a life that I knew. It was quite a "cattle call" of wheelchairs when they pushed us all out there, but we sure appreciated it.

Of course, I got quite a few gifts during the time I was hospitalized, and one of the neatest things that I got was a "countdown box." It consisted of 14 little gifts on the ends of strings. So every day for 14 days, after I had finished my therapy, I would pull the string, and I'd have a little gift. That really gave me something to look forward to. And I always looked forward to my mom's visits. She came every day and chatted with me, and if it was a nice day, she would push my wheelchair out on the sun porch. We prayed together a lot, and by that time in my life, I already had a very strong faith in a personal Savior. I really cherished that faith because it helped me center my thoughts on the fact that I wasn't alone in this process and that God would be with me.

It was sometime in the middle of September that I got to go home. If I remember correctly, I went home in walking casts. The casts extended from about mid-calf level to up above my knees. They had cut a strip down the middle of them, and there were holes over my kneecaps, so there would be some flexibility. I was able to walk and get around the house a little, but only with great care.

I remember that when they cut the holes in that cast, they were using what seemed, at least through the eyes of a child, to be a huge saw. Of course, I was reassured that there would be no problem, but I did notice that the people doing the cutting seemed pretty young, so I was rather apprehensive. Well, my apprehension was justified. The saw slipped and cut my kneecap. It wasn't a deep cut, but I saw the blood, and that greatly affected my perceptions of the credibility of the people doing the cutting! Believe me; I thought about that incident every time thereafter when a saw was used to cut one of my casts.

After I was released from the hospital, I just stayed at home for a while. The school provided me with a tutor, so I wouldn't get too far behind on my studies. It wasn't until some time in December that I finally returned to school so that I could finish the fourth grade. By that time, I had been fitted with a back brace because I was already starting to develop a scoliosis. The brace wasn't too uncomfortable.

I believe that I wore a body sock under it, and my clothes fit over it, so it wasn't that noticeable.

I had some continuing physical therapy for a while as an outpatient. I think that I had the therapy twice a week, at least at first, and I had exercises that I had to do at home. My mom helped me do those exercises every day. I remember that I'd lie on the floor and try to do leg lifts and scissors kicks. I think I was also supposed to sit on the edge of a table or bed and lift up my legs, but that was a lost cause. The idea behind the exercises was that, unless they were totally dead, nerve endings could be reactivated. If they were totally dead, however, they would not come back. Unfortunately, that apparently was the case with many of the nerve endings in my legs.

I'm sure the whole ordeal of my hospitalization and then my therapy was very difficult for my mom, but she was a trooper through it all. Whatever the doctors said to do, she did. If somebody had a home remedy that sounded reasonable and wouldn't interfere with anything that was already being done, she'd try that as well. I remember mom heard that rubbing cocoa butter on the muscles activated them, so she got some cocoa butter, and we tried it. It didn't work, but getting a massage with cocoa butter probably couldn't have done any harm.

Another way my mom helped me was by not being overprotective. She allowed me to do things that I don't believe I would have allowed my child to do. Now, I believe that children should be reared to "fly" on their own, but I don't know if I would have had as much courage as my mother. She just put that walking cast on me and sent me out there to try most anything. I even tried riding my bike with those casts on my legs. I probably didn't get very far, but mom let me try it. She never said, "Oh, you're too sick to try that." Instead, she allowed me to discover on my own what I could or couldn't do, and I will be forever grateful for that.

Even with my therapy, exercises, and family encouragement, I was left with some residual effects that just weren't going to go away. The worst of these was my scoliosis, so we were referred to an orthopedic physician at Abbott Northwestern Hospital in Minneapolis. It was just called Northwestern Hospital at that time. This particular physician had an excellent track record with spinal fusion. He also had this idea about transplanting tendons from the upper part of my legs and criss-crossing them over my stomach and attaching them to my rib cage and hip bones. Since my stomach muscles no longer functioned, the transplanted tendons would take their place and give my trunk some support. So, between fifth and sixth grade, I was back in the hospital having tendon transplant surgery.

The surgery was done in August, and of course, it was beastly hot again. To make matters worse, I was under 12, so I had to be on the children's ward. I'm the youngest in my family, and I never spent a lot of time around babies. There I was on a ward with all of these babies that cried all night. I thought I was going to go **mad**. In addition to the noise, I had to lie on my back. I had always slept on my side or my stomach, so I just couldn't sleep at all. I had pillows under my knees, and I had to stay in this sort of folded-envelope position, and it was so hot and sticky. I'd finally fall asleep at two or three in the morning, and then one of those babies would start to cry and wake me up. It was one of the worst times in my life. I can remember lying there for three or four weeks and just waiting for the time to pass, and it finally did.

The surgery was successful in that the tendon transplant took and healed well. However, as far as function, it wasn't particularly successful unless you always intend to inhale. When you breathe in, the rib cage pulls back. But you also have to exhale. Because of that, my surgeon recommended that I always wear a stiff girdle for support, and I have. However, that hasn't always been easy. Girdles were not in style then, and if you're a size 8 or 10 as I am, heavy, paneled-front girdles are difficult to find.

I got out of the hospital in time to start the fifth grade that fall, and I was actually able to spend that whole year in school. However, my scoliosis was getting progressively more severe and now had become an "S" curve. I had been going to a chiropractor, and he did electrotherapy and had used other types of treatment to try and correct the situation, but none of it worked. My folks always involved me in decisions regarding my treatment, and I remember them telling me that my scoliosis wasn't going to get any better unless I had spinal fusion surgery. They also told me that I would need to be put in a body cast for a couple of months before the surgery could be performed. It seemed that there was no other alternative, so during January of 1956, when I was in the sixth grade, I had to withdraw from school again in order to begin the body cast procedure.

Having the body cast put on was quite an ordeal. I remember that they strapped my head in this contraption and dangled me off the floor during the entire process of fitting and molding that cast. It took about three hours, and it was grueling and exhausting. To make matters worse, they fashioned that first cast to be something like a torture chamber. It went from above my chin to down past my hips. They wanted me to stretch out the curvature of the spine, so I couldn't eat unless I lifted my chin up over the top of the cast. That way I would stretch out my spine every time I ate. It was terribly uncomfortable. Fortunately, I wasn't claustrophobic, or I don't think I could have stood living in that cast.

I had my first back surgery in April of 1956. They cut a long window in the back of the cast and operated through that window. The procedure took about four or five hours and involved chipping out pieces of pelvic bone and inserting them between the vertebrae. I think the first surgery fused the lower part of my spine, and during the second one, they did the upper part. The procedure was the same for the second surgery as it was for the first; pieces of bone were again chipped from my pelvis and wedged between the vertebrae, but this time in the upper regions of the spine.

There was about a four-week wait between the first and second surgeries, and I had to stay in the hospital the whole time. It was quite a long hospitalization, but my mom stayed down in the Twin Cities, at least during the time I was recuperating from the surgeries, so I got to see her every day; that helped a lot.

I can remember lamenting the fact that I would always be embarrassed to wear a swimming suit because the scar on my back would be visible. As it turned out, the scar really isn't bad. In fact, it's barely noticeable. It was such a clean incision that it just left a fine line. I have a much bigger scar on my hip where they took the pieces of bone out. But the scars have never really been a problem.

I got out of the hospital in late May or early June, but I still wasn't able to get out of bed. I had to stay in a hospital bed that had been put in the middle of the dining room because we couldn't fit that big bed into my bedroom. The plan was that I would stay flat on my back in bed until November, and then I would be able to get up and get on with my life. However, it just so happened that before I left the hospital, the body cast had been lightened a little in the pelvic area so that it would be easier for me to maneuver on and off of bed pans. Unfortunately, they lightened it too much, and it cracked, which allowed for some pelvic movement. I knew right away that something was wrong. I could feel it, so I told my mom, and she called the doctor.

Getting me back and forth to the hospital was really involved. We had a two door 1955 Chevy, and for me to get in, the back of the seat on the rider's side had to be removed. A board was then slid in, and I would have to lie on top of that board. Mom sat in the back seat next to me. It worked out fine, but it was somewhat of an ordeal. Also, dad was the foreman of his business, and it was difficult for him to take time off of work, so I only went to the hospital when it was absolutely necessary. The doctor knew how difficult it was for my parents to get me down to the Twin Cities, so he suggested that my mom just patch the cast herself, and that's what she did.

The day was finally approaching when I was to go to the hospital and get my cast replaced and, hopefully, get approval to get back on my feet again. Even though it was going to be another several hour ordeal, I was so anxious for that day to arrive. I remember the week before that was to happen; I was lying there thinking, "Boy, I wish it was next Monday. This would all be over." Unfortunately, however, I learned something that week in November of 1956 that has shaped my life. I will **never** wish my life away again. For the rest of my life, I will never wish it's a month from now, or a week from now, or even a day from now. Because when we got down to the hospital, the doctor discovered that when the cast had cracked, the fusion had slipped and hadn't healed correctly. So the day I had wished for so fervently had finally arrived, but instead of being back on my feet, I was back in the hospital having a third surgery on my back!

After that surgery, I was back in bed, and there were more casts, of course. I didn't get up and out of bed until some time in April of 1957. I had been confined to bed for an entire year, and when I was finally told I could get up, my feet were numb, and I could no longer walk. I guess after a year in bed, we should have expected that. However, the doctors never said anything about that possibility. Had they told my parents to massage my feet or do any other therapy, they certainly would have followed directions. But they were never told to do anything with my feet, and now I was unable to walk. So after all that, it seemed like we were back to square one. I have never seen my dad as discouraged as he was at that moment.

We had come through four or five years of therapy, exercises, surgeries, braces, casts, going two steps forward and one step back, and now I had to learn to walk all over again. So my parents got me the kitchen chair, and I started to push it around the house. The chair slid across the floor pretty easily, and that's how I learned to walk the third time.

As my spinal fusion healed and became sturdier, the doctors

gradually started to cut down the size of my cast. Those little saws were back, but this time I didn't mind. They first cut the cast down so it was just around my neck and upper body; then it was cut so that it resembled a strapless swimsuit. And that fall, the sides were cut out and straps attached so that I could take it off when I went to bed. What a glorious feeling that was! After spending a year and a half in a body cast, I remember feeling the sheets against my skin and thinking, "Hey! This is nice stuff." It was during January of 1958 that I was finally able to go about my daily life without the cast. I had first been put in a body cast in January of 1956, so I was encased in plaster for a total of two years!

I had gone back to school in October of 1957 while I was still wearing the cast. Since I had received homebound instruction for my entire seventh-grade year, I had few friends at school anymore. I knew some kids with whom I had gone to elementary school, but they were hardly elated to see me again. I'm told that the other children were cruel to me. I don't remember any specific incidents, but I do remember feeling weird and awkward. I got a lot of support from my family, but I remember feeling very much like a "loner" at school. I think that was probably a pretty accurate perception. My schoolmates were all painfully aware that I was different.

I felt slow and awkward, especially going up or down stairs. I went to Central Junior High School, which is now City Hall, and those grand stairs were quite a care, particularly with the added weight of the body cast. Of course, that was long before there were any concerns about handicapped accessibility. It was handicapped accessible if you could access it. I could, but only with great care.

Even when I wasn't on the stairs, I always walked very slowly, and people would just walk away from me. Eighth grade turned out to be a fairly rugged year for me. I started to vomit up blood in February, and to this day, I'm not exactly sure why, though I would suppose that I had an ulcer. I assume that I was having some kind of a nervous reaction to the trauma of finally being plunged back into the real world and not having it go all that well. It's hard enough just being 14, but wearing a body cast really complicates things.

Because of the symptoms I was experiencing, I was hospitalized and given all sorts of tests that required drinking this awful tasting stuff. However, they never found a cause for my vomiting. I think that I received a miracle from the Lord. I was praying as were many others, and our prayers were answered. All they found was that my blood count was low, which certainly didn't come as any big surprise, so I was given liver shots. I'd already had more than my share of shots, but those liver shots were incredible. It felt like the needle was as big around as my finger!

After I was released from this latest hospitalization, I returned to school, and things started to go much better for me. By this time, the cast was gone, and I no longer thought of myself as handicapped. I did, or at least tried, virtually anything the other kids my age did. I wore three-inch spike heels; I even tried skiing, but I wasn't very good at it. My legs went in opposite directions. I couldn't run or jump, but I was able to do most of the things I wanted to do. So, beginning with the spring of 1958, I was able to live a pretty normal life once again. I graduated from high school in 1962, went to college, married, and have had a wonderful career as a music teacher. This is my 29th year, and I wish everyone could enjoy their work the way that I enjoy mine.

Over the years, of course, I have seen physicians about my spinal fusion and other polio-related matters, but it's no longer easy to find a physician who knows much about polio and its effects. Virtually all the physicians who knew of our conditions and what we've been through are retired or deceased, so it behooves every one of us to find a specialist with the expertise to deal with our situations. I saw the surgeon who did my spinal fusion shortly before he retired. When I asked him for a referral to another orthopedic specialist, he just said, "All I can say to you is that I really don't have anyone to whom I can refer you. I would suggest that since you've gotten along as well as you have, I certainly wouldn't do anything drastic."

I did go to the Scoliosis Clinic in Minneapolis in 1980. A couple of years before that I had wrenched my lower back, and by trying to favor it, apparently I had damaged the disk immediately below the fusion. One of the doctors there was testing my knees looking for reflexes, and he discovered I didn't have any. He looked over at the other physician in the examining room and said, "She did walk in here; didn't she?" The other doctor looked at him and said, "Yeah, but I'm not sure how." I guess I wasn't a textbook case, and that's the real challenge of post-polio residuals; everyone's case is unique.

About the only suggestion they had for me was that I should have a little more support for my stomach, so they sent me over to be fitted for a brace. I thought, "Here we go again." They fitted me with this contraption that looked a little like something made of left-over parts from the hospital's padded-cell section. It was so bulky that it threw off my balance. I felt awful in it. I did try to wear it for a few weeks, but eventually it ended up in the closet. After that experience, for the next several years, I was just more or less my own doctor.

Recently though, over the last few years, I've been having increased joint and muscle pain, and I knew that I needed to see someone about my situation. My general practitioner suggested that I go to Sister Kenny Institute in Minneapolis, and it took him about five years to convince me to do so. I guess I was afraid they were going to tell me I had to withdraw from life. Finally, in March of 1992, I did go there for a post-polio evaluation. I had an appointment with Dr. Richard Owen who evaluated my muscle functioning. I also saw a physical therapist and had a stress test. I learned which of my muscles are weak, and I was given some exercises that are aerobic in nature but won't make me overtired. I also learned that I need to be very careful not to push myself to the point of exhaustion. In my case, if I work my muscles too hard, I will fall. If I don't pay for overdoing immediately by falling, I'll pay for it in the future by having to use braces or a wheelchair. That's a pretty severe message, but most of us will take that chance. We think that we can do all the things that we used to do and still want to do, but if we do those things too often, then we're going to lose that gamble. And now, in 1994, I'm having to accept the fact that I will need an electric cart to continue my career in teaching.

I've known the feelings coming from people (real or imagined) of pity, and I wonder if they are thinking, "I wish these handicapped people would get out of the way." Maybe I think too much about things like that, but people's opinions have always been important to me, and I have learned in many different ways that it is all right to be handicapped if people don't have to accommodate you.

I believe that the hardest thing for me now is to realize that all of the thought processes that helped me overcome my handicap, the attitudes of, "If it's painful, I'll work through it; if it's hard, I'll work harder. If there's a task to be done, I'll do it; I don't need any help," no longer apply. That's the attitude that keeps you driving through your therapy to overcome your handicap. And now, in this part of my life, I have to find a way to accept that if I don't work from seven in the morning to midnight, I'm still valuable. And that's the hardest lesson of all, because so much of my life has been serving and living up to people's expectations. And now I have to say, "How can I live within my limitations and still be the same person I was?" And that's difficult for me.

I have clear memories of my first therapist in the hospital. She didn't want a whimper or a tear from any of us. We were to be tough and gritty. I did what was expected. I didn't question, and I got well! These were my strongest memories of the lessons I had learned. I needed to have a disciplined life with a no-quit attitude. That was what worked. But it doesn't work for me anymore. Now, I am learning that I must rest when I'm tired. To work through the point of pain has caused muscle damage. However, people's expectations of me (morning meetings, bus duty after a full teaching day, obligations such as concerts/weddings) and my own desire to be part of life's mainstream, combined with my stubborn "I can do it myself" attitude, tend to keep me from putting the limitations on my schedule that I should.

The basic problem is that I still really have trouble seeing myself as handicapped. My husband finally convinced me that I should apply for a handicapped parking permit, and you would think that my need for handicapped parking would be easy for me to accept. Well, think again! When I went into the Drivers' License Bureau to be interviewed for the permit, I was really feeling low. I didn't like asking for special privileges, nor did I want to disclose that it is sometimes hard for me to walk. I also expected them to look at me incredulously, "You're handicapped?" I just knew they were going to think I was trying to pull a fast one.

Even now when I pull into a handicapped parking space and see people looking at me as if I'm just faking it, my thinking varies from wanting to limp a lot so they will turn away and leave me alone to wanting to look up at them and smile. I am not paranoid; I know they look. One day at Crossroads Shopping Center, a man called out to me from across the parking lot, "Are you really handicapped?" I was really hurting that day, and I was so angry with him for challenging me. I looked up at him and said in a loud, direct voice, "Yes sir, I really am!" He turned and walked off, and I think I cried a little. I wish I would have said, "Yes I am, and on behalf of all of us who are, thank you for helping police these spots."

In spite of my polio, no one in my family ever thought of me as handicapped until recently when I had to disclose that I was unable to do certain things I used to do, like go for walks after family dinners. My family is great to get out and walk, but now I find I need to spare my muscles that kind of pastime. My sister Lois was in a dinner meeting a few years ago, and when people were asked to raise their hands if they had a family member who was handicapped, Lois didn't raise her hand. When she told me about this, she added,

"I guess I have never thought of you as handicapped." That really didn't surprise me because until recently, I have never thought of myself as handicapped either.

However, even before I had anyone tell me that my disability was going to require me to do some adaptive living, I've been doing it. Very few people, including myself, ever realized what kind of mental gymnastics I would go through when, during some activity, we would come to a place where people were going up or down hills or staircases, and I would have to decide the adaptive method of doing that. I recently discovered that even I often don't realize all of the things I have to do to accomplish something that a non-handicapped person does without any special effort. I guess I have had these various disabilities so long that I truly don't know what it feels like to have the full capabilities of all my muscles. I was a runner as a child; I truly loved to run. I loved racing, and I was good at it. After polio I would occasionally have dreams about running, and I could feel the sensation in my mind. I no longer have any recall of what it feels like to run, and I grieve that a little. I would like to remember the sensation of running and the joy that it brought me. However, even walking is hard for me now. So on good days when I feel strong, I enjoy walking in much the same way that I used to enjoy running.

I am the most nervous about walking in crowds. I know that if someone bumped me behind one of my knees or pushed me a little, I would probably fall down, causing injury and embarrassment. I have no knee reflexes and very little lift for my feet at the ankles. I compensate for that by lifting my foot with my big toe. If I understand it correctly, the extender part of each leg muscle is almost normal, whereas the reflex part of the same muscle is almost non-existent. This causes the muscle to fight to stabilize, and results in some pain.

I fall now and then, usually in sets of three, and just why it happens is a little involved. I find that if I have not had enough sleep, (less than six hours) and if my schedule is pressure packed, I really can't expect to hurry and rush around without stumbling and falling. If I say to myself, "You must be careful; you are on a tightrope," I can avoid it; however, when you are really busy, it is sometimes hard to remember to coach yourself by silently chanting, "Remember to lift your left foot. Remember to lift your left foot..."

Some of my falls recently have damaged my hands, and I am really concerned about my hands. This is true, not just because I play harp and piano, but because I so greatly need my right hand for the railings that get me up and down stairs. Even as early as 12 years ago, I realized that a house with a lot of stairs would be extremely hard for me to be comfortable in. When we looked at houses, we specified that it should be a one story. That has turned out to be a good decision.

In 1991 I made a discovery that hardwood floors or cement create a lot of discomfort in my bones and give me joint pain. I had suspected as much during the 1990-91 school year when I moved to South Junior High School, and my classroom floor was tile over concrete. I hurt so much I wanted to scream by midday. I asked for a carpet on the lower level of my three-tier room. I even offered to buy it, but the school district found a piece of carpet that would make a fair sized area rug and put it in. That helped, but I have a tendency to drag that left toe, so I occasionally have fallen because of the rug. The comfort in my bones has made it worth the risk, but I really wish they had let me fund this effort so I could have what I really needed. Recently, my husband Bill and I carpeted the kitchen, and we went with a thicker rug, and a thicker padding just for comfort for my body. This has made a big, positive difference.

I have learned to pace myself. If I do a little housework and a little shopping on Saturdays, that is far better than doing all the shopping or all the housework. Staying too long at any one physically demanding activity increases my pain. I need to partner standing and walking activities with sitting down activities, and I have to keep exploring appropriate sitting and walking techniques as well as the right chairs and shoes.

My doctor at Sister Kenny Institute has helped me a great deal. She, like several doctors I've seen over the last 15 years, thinks that I'm in pretty good shape for the shape I'm in, and that encourages me to give God the glory for the great things He has done. There were some people who told my mom I probably wouldn't walk again, but my mother didn't believe that, and I never heard it. Together we teamed up to do extensive therapy which brought me to the place I am today. I know I am in need of an appropriate mind-set, and so holding close to me the faith in God that has made the difference in how I felt about life and its challenges, I want to mold the attitude of winning, and shape that into something practical that will work for me and the people I love.

Chapter 6

Braces, Crutches, and Canes

Many of those we interviewed have worn braces or needed the assistance of crutches or canes at some point in their lives. Those such as Len Jordan and Arvid Schwartz have worn a brace of some sort since their acute illness. Others who originally needed a brace or crutches recovered sufficiently to walk without assistance. Some continue to do so. However, those like Diane Keyser and Mary Ann Hoffman, who are experiencing polio's late effects, have had to return to the use of braces, crutches, or other aids for ambulation. For some, such as Diane Keyser, a return to the use of such aids has been a difficult adjustment. Others, like Mary Ann Hoffman, have accepted the need for aid with ambulation more easily. In fact, Mary Ann makes a fashion statement with her crutches!

Though the use of braces, crutches, or canes is a common feature of these stories, they include a great deal more. As was the case with the other chapters, the stories are included in their entirety.

Len Jordan

Some time in late July of 1945, when I was 10 years old, I suffered an injury while jumping off the back of a truck. It wasn't a serious injury, but my leg and back were pretty sore. I had thought that the pain would start to go away after a couple of days, but it didn't. Instead, it started getting worse, particularly my back pain. It got to the point that the left side of my back and my hip were hurting so badly that my aunt started putting hot towels on me, sort of like Sister Kenny did with polio patients, just to help alleviate some of my pain. But the pain still didn't go away, and within about five days, I actually started losing the use of my one leg. The leg would just sort of go out on me, and I would fall down.

I was living with my Aunt Lydia and Uncle Karl at that time. I had lost my dad when I was eight, and my mom had lost custody of me. My aunt was getting quite worried, so she called the doctor, but he just kept telling her that he didn't think it was anything too serious. Nobody thought about the possibility that I had polio because I didn't have a fever or any other symptoms except for the back pain and the problem with my leg. But I just kept getting worse and worse, and finally it was decided that I needed to go to the hospital.

My oldest cousin, Jordy, had to carry me out to the car, and then they took me to Swedish Hospital in downtown Minneapolis. I spent the next two days there, and our family doctor, as well as the staff at Swedish Hospital, couldn't figure out what was wrong with me. Eventually, somebody decided that I should have a spinal tap, so about two full weeks after I first started to have symptoms, I was finally diagnosed with polio.

Right after the diagnosis was made, I was transferred to Sister Kenny Institute in Minneapolis. They put me into a contagion ward where I couldn't have any visitors. I must have spent about three weeks in that ward, and then they moved me upstairs. I got the treatments with the hot packs at Sister Kenny Institute, and because of those treatments, the polio finally stopped spreading just short of my hip. The whole leg was affected, and I did have a little bit of paralysis in my left upper arm. My heart and lungs were never affected though, and my right side was okay, which is a good thing because I'm right-handed.

I was hospitalized for a total of 11 months. However, I was only at the main site of the Sister Kenny Institute for about three of those months. Everything seemed to happen on the 13th of the month. I went into the Kenny Institute on August 13, 1945, and I got out on July 13, 1946. During that time, of course, I had a great deal of therapy. I remember doing many, many sit-ups and touching my toes a lot. I still try to do that, touch my toes, but now something seems to get in the way!

I have some real clear memories of my stay at Sister Kenny Institute. A couple of us were sort of "roust-abouts." We would run around in our wheelchairs after hours, causing problems and chasing the nurses. We wouldn't have known what to do with them if we had caught them, but we sure had fun trying. When you're hospitalized that long, you have to do something to break the monotony.

Fortunately, they did do some things to entertain us and keep us busy. I remember that we had puppet shows and other entertainment. We also did all sorts of arts and crafts like pillow making and fly-tying. After I was out of isolation, I had a lot of visitors. My mom came sometimes; though like I said, by that time she had already lost custody of me. And occasionally one of my sisters would come. Mostly, though, it was my aunt and uncle and their kids who visited me. They had become sort of my step-family.

I think that my aunt and uncle felt a lot of responsibility for my getting polio, though of course, it sure wasn't their fault. They were both very loving people and gave me a lot of attention. My aunt was more the one to give me hugs and kisses. My uncle was a rather stern man, but yet he was very kind to me. He even made a couple of toys for me at the machine shop where he worked.

Compared to the other people at Sister Kenny, I tended to be one of the lucky ones in that I wasn't completely bedridden. I was able to get into a wheelchair after a relatively short period of time. A little later, I was trained to use the Kenny crutches with the straps, and I ended up using two of those crutches for a couple of years.

I actually met Sister Kenny twice during my hospitalization. She would come through the ward and occasionally stop and talk with us. I remember her very well. I can still see her face, the heavyset features, the gray hair. She was a pretty stout old gal, maybe 5'11" or so, and well over 200 pounds. Yet, she was a beautiful woman, both inside and outside. She had a way about her that was very smooth. She carried herself well, and just looking at her you got a feeling that she knew what she was doing. I probably still have her autograph somewhere, though I'm not sure if I could find it.

Like I said earlier, I was only at Sister Kenny Institute for about three months. The epidemic was very bad that year, and they needed the space out there for the newer cases, so I was moved out to Fort Snelling. I guess they were using any facility around the Twin Cities that they could find, because that place (Fort Snelling) was terrible. We were put in the Army barracks out there, and they were dark and dreary, kind of like a dungeon. It was a terrifying place for a child to have to stay.

Fortunately, I only spent about two weeks there. Then they transferred me over to the Navy barracks at Chamberlain Airport.

That was much better. It was a wider and brighter building, and the walls were white, not brown like they were at Fort Snelling. Also, we had some entertainment there, and I gained the favor of a couple of the Navy guys, so they would take me to see a movie or to the base PX.

All total, I ended up spending 11 months in four different places, and I'm sure my hospital bills were huge. Even back then in the 1940's, if I remember correctly, the hospital bill was somewhere between $50,000 and $60,000. However, Sister Kenny and the March of Dimes covered everything. My aunt and uncle just had an average income, plus they had three kids of their own to take care of, so I don't know how they would have ever been able to pay a bill like that. Because of how much they helped me, I've always donated to the March of Dimes and Sister Kenny Institute. They'll always have a special place in my heart.

When I was finally released from the hospital, I was still walking with two crutches which, of course, hampered my ability to compete with the other boys in sports and things. I was able to eventually get rid of both of those crutches when I was about 15 or so. I was pretty self-conscious when I first got out of the hospital, so I just stayed home and played in the house a lot. But when I started getting my motors back, I was able to overcome some of my self-consciousness, and then I got out more and tried to play most games the other kids were playing.

Even after I no longer had to use my crutches for walking, I'd sometimes use one of them when I'd run. Because of that, I got two different nicknames as a kid. One was "Hop-a-long," and the other was "Step-and-a-half." That's still my handle today, "Step-and-a-half." Of course, back then, I didn't always like being called those nicknames. I was pretty self-conscious about how I looked and how I walked. I guess I still am. When I walk with people or when I go to a swimming pool, I know that people are staring at me, but I think we all tend to look at each other no matter what. So if they do, I guess it's no big deal.

Getting back to when I was a kid, I was lucky in that I had two or three friends from the neighborhood who really stuck by me, and we'd play together with our toy trucks, cars, or trains. However, I was able to do only about half of the sports activities that the other kids were doing. I always tried to do things, but a lot of times I couldn't do them very well, or I couldn't do the whole activity. For instance, when we'd play kick the can, I would kick it, but somebody else would run for me. That was the same way I played baseball; they'd let me hit, but then someone else would have to run the bases. I also loved to play football, and though I couldn't run, I had a pretty good throwing arm.

I even got a bicycle after I had polio. I must have been 13 or 14 years old when I bought it from one of my cousins. I don't think I owned a bicycle before my polio, but I got that bike while I was still using my crutches, and I had to get on a step and sort of push myself off. I gradually got to the point where I could even pump a little bit with my left leg. I rode that bike so that I could get to places that I had trouble walking to like Sunday school. Sometimes I even rode it to school, but usually I walked. It was a seven block walk, and I did it twice a day, because I came home for lunch. Even though I would walk as fast as I could, I was usually the last one home. But it didn't matter, I still managed to get there eventually.

Believe it or not, I actually got a letter for sports in high school. The coach asked me to try out for football. I could throw the ball a long way, and the boys always liked me to play quarterback because I threw the ball so well. I was the second farthest thrower in the school, but I couldn't run, and I really couldn't do a lot of the things that you needed to do to play on the team, so I never went out for football. I knew I'd get killed. Instead, I was just the manager of the baseball team, and I got a letter for keeping score and taking care of the equipment and stuff. Even though I didn't really play on the team, that letter still meant a lot to me.

After I finished 10th grade, I went to Dunwoody Industrial Institute and learned to be a printer. I was very fortunate in that the state of Minnesota not only paid for my schooling, but they also gave me a little money for transportation and room and board. I became a linotype operator, then went into graphic sales and ownership, which gave me a very good career. And I think that my having a good trade that allowed me to be self-supporting was the whole point of the state helping me with my education. I paid them back many times over by becoming a productive, tax-paying citizen.

In addition to having a successful career, I led a very normal home and family life. I was married, had four children, and now have seven grandchildren. My wife died of cancer in 1985, and after being alone for 10 years, I am now planning to remarry.

I did have to have a couple of surgeries because of my polio. The first one was done in 1952 when I was 19 years old. The idea was to fix my ankle so that the foot wouldn't drop any more. There's a little play in the ankle, but not much. Ever since I had polio, that foot has never been of much use to me. I've never been able to move the toes very much, and really, from the knee down, it's pretty much useless. My left leg is an inch and a half shorter, so I wear a built-up shoe to compensate.

I went into Gillette Hospital in St. Paul, where they operated on me. They froze my ankle by inserting stainless steel pins and scraping the cartilage. They also put staples on the right side of it. The surgery fused my ankle at almost a 90 degree angle, so I no longer have a drop foot, but it was years before I overcame the pain that operation caused me. As a matter of fact, it still hurts when I touch my ankle, and the surgery was done over 40 years ago!

My second surgery was done in 1973. At that time, I had what they called a "Great Jones and hammer toe operation." I needed that surgery because my right foot, which is my "good" foot, had taken such a pounding over the years. After all, I've led a very active life. I've gone hiking and the whole bit, and I've always put most of my weight on the right leg, so I needed to get those toes fixed up. And right now, I have another toe that needs some work to be done, so I suppose I'll need to have a third surgery pretty soon.

I've also worn leg braces over the years. The one brace that I wore for many years was just for my ankle, and it would hold my foot up. It basically consisted of a leather strap and a steel spring. I would put it on over an old sock, and then I'd put my regular sock and shoe on over it. The spring would break from time to time, but I would just replace it.

In 1981, I went into what they call an "Iowa" knee brace. It went about halfway up the thigh and halfway down the calf. I wore that until about 1987 or 1988, and then I went into a full leg brace that has what they call an off-center hinge. The hinge forces my knee back when my heel comes into contact with the ground. The brace fits into my shoe. Putting the shoe on can sometimes present quite a challenge, so I have to use a shoe horn to squeeze my foot into the shoe.

Even now that I'm wearing the long leg brace, I still fall down two or three times a week. The problem is that the knee just gives out, and there's a point where, if the brace doesn't lock itself soon enough, then on the next step, I'll go down. Because of that, I walk with my hand on my leg, and I've started using a cane again for stability. I realize, though, that I need to get a better brace, and now with my Medicare and disability benefits, I'm going to look into getting a brace with rubber assists on the hinges that will give me a little better control.

It's interesting, but even with my limp and all the braces I've worn over the years, people usually don't have any idea what's wrong with my leg. They never seem to think that my limp is from polio. Instead, they think that I broke my leg or something. For instance, I remember one printing customer that I had been calling on for over a year. Finally, he noticed my limp and said, "Well, what happened to you? Did you hurt yourself over the weekend?" I said, "Do you really want to know?" And he did want to know, so I told him. But most people don't really care about anyone else's problems, so they usually don't ask.

Lately though, particularly since I've been using a cane, people are more likely to notice that I have a disability, and so they'll often open doors for me and give me other sorts of help. I don't really like getting a lot of help as I've been very independent all of my life. I've ridden horses, portaged canoes, flown airplanes, but now it's getting to the point where I realize that I need some help from time to time, so I'm starting to accept it better.

I guess that it's really been these last 10 years or so that I've kind of gone downhill. I've started to have quite a bit of back pain, and I'm afraid to do some things because I think I might fall or injure my back. My leg has also gotten weaker. It was never very good, but now I think it's down to about only one or two percent of normal strength, at least from the knee down. I've gotten several opinions about it from different people, and at least three orthopedic doctors have told me that the motor in the knee has just worn itself out. So my leg tires very easily, and I have to rest it more often. Surprisingly, it tends to give me as much trouble lying down as it does when I'm walking, so I end up shifting around in bed quite a bit in order to get comfortable.

With the decline of strength in my leg and because of the problems that I have with my left hip and lower back, I have a lot of trouble doing some of the things that I used to do. I do as much for myself as I can, though. I still do maintenance things around the house, but I know that I have to pace myself. For instance, I painted the house recently. I climbed up on the ladder and everything, but after doing so, I needed to take a few days off to rest and sit in the whirlpool. I've learned that I need to take care of myself and stay within my limits. As long as I keep doing that, I think things will be just fine.

Mary Ann Hoffman

I was raised on a farm in Foster County of east central North Dakota. During late summer of 1947, I was 10 years old and looking forward to taking a trip with my grandparents who lived with us on the farm. They were going to take me to Buffalo, New York, and we were going to visit our relatives there. However, I came down with polio, so I never got to make the trip.

I remember that my symptoms started on the Sunday before we were going to leave. I was a very active child, and that day I had been out in the barn, roller skating up in the hay loft. I came in and told my parents that I was feeling sick, and my muscles ached. I had a terrible headache and a temperature, so my mother told me to lie down.

By Tuesday of that week, I was still very sick. However, I was hoping I'd get better in time to leave with my grandparents, so mother went to town and bought me some new clothes for the trip. I didn't get better though, and I remember feeling devastated when my grandparents had to leave without me.

Sometime that week, our family doctor came out to the house to examine me. He thought that I had rheumatic fever. I also remember that he looked in my throat and said, "Those tonsils need to come out. As soon as you get over this, we'll put you in the hospital and take them out." Well, I've still got those tonsils. They were all right, but I wasn't! Shortly after the doctor's visit, I started to have trouble walking. When I'd try to get up, my legs would just collapse out from under me.

I don't remember everything that happened, but I know that within a few days, I was taken to St. Luke's Hospital in Fargo. The evening that I went in, my dad was out harvesting. It must have been about 9:00 P.M. by the time he got back to the house, and he and mom talked it over and decided that we needed to go to Fargo. One of our friends had a small airport in McHenry, so we went over there, and I was flown to Fargo. I was then taken by ambulance to the hospital, where they did a spinal tap. Within minutes, I was diagnosed with polio. After the diagnosis, I was immediately put into the isolation ward. The doctors told my father that I would be in isolation for at least two weeks, so he might as well go home because he wouldn't be allowed to see me.

So in I went, into a private room on the first floor of the hospital. I remember it as being a rather small room, down on the corner of the hall. Though I couldn't have visitors, I was lucky in that the husband of my mother's first cousin (I called him "Uncle Lyle") was an administrator at St. Luke's. When I started being a little more coherent, he'd come and sit outside my door to talk to me and keep me company. For the whole time I was in isolation, Uncle Lyle was the only member of my family with whom I had any contact.

After a couple of weeks, I was moved to a different room. I had a little baby boy or girl, I'm not sure which, as a roommate for a while. The baby was eventually moved to the pediatric ward, but I never went to pediatrics. Instead, I stayed in that room until my release from the hospital, which was probably in May. Since I entered the hospital around the beginning of September, I must have been there for a total of about nine months.

My parents came to visit me whenever they could, and I even had a visit from my best friend, Marlys. I think she came to see me over the Thanksgiving holiday. However, they wouldn't allow her to come up to my room. Rather, I was brought down to the main entrance, and we had to visit there. Even though I had been out of isolation for quite some time, they kept us about 20 feet apart, and we almost had to yell at each other to be heard. People were coming and going through the lobby, and Marlys's parents and a nurse were there, so we had no privacy. Marlys looked like she was going to cry the whole time, but I tried to put up a brave front. Though I had been really excited about her visit, it turned out to be a disappointing experience.

I did get to go home for one visit. I think I was supposed to go home for Christmas, but I had a bronchial infection, so I didn't get to go. Instead, I went in maybe January or February. Though I'm not sure of the date, I know it was cold out, and there was snow on the ground. We flew home in an airplane with skis so we could land right at our farm. That was kind of exciting.

As far as my stay at the hospital, I think that I adjusted pretty well. Not that I enjoyed it, but I think I just made the best of it. I remember there was a young fellow in the room across the hall, and once I started feeling better, I would play checkers and cards with him. That helped to pass the time. I also remember that I had a tutor who came once a week to give me my school lessons. Of course, I was supposed to work on those lessons a little every day, but instead I did them a couple of hours before the tutor got there!

I also did some "creative" things while I was in the hospital. For instance, I had the hot-pack machine in my room. It was an old-time washing machine with a wringer. I looked at that thing every day and wondered what would happen if I took the hose off. Well, one day I just decided to try it, and away went the water, all over the floor! I also used to shoot spit balls and stick them to the ceiling. Eventually, they'd dry out and fall off, but one time while I was doing that the head nurse came into my room to see me. Fortunately, she didn't look up at the ceiling, but after she left my room, I got an aide and said, "Get me a broom. We've got to get those spit balls down before she comes back!"

Another thing that I did to entertain myself was to race my wheelchair. We had the old style wheelchairs with the big wheels in the front, but you could really maneuver those things. A boy from Fargo and I used to race our wheelchairs down this long ramp, but one time I was trying to pass him on the curve, and my wheelchair tipped over. I wasn't hurt, but that ended my career as a wheelchair racer.

Other than those things, I guess I pretty much behaved myself. However, I always had a lot of energy and wanted to get up and go, so when they let me get back in a wheelchair, I'd go down and sit at the front door of the hospital. I'd drink cokes and watch the visitors come and go. Sometimes I'd play tic-tac-toe with the nurses. I was a champion at that.

As far as my medical treatment, for a while I got the heat treatment in order to reduce my muscle tightness. I didn't have a whole lot of muscle tightness, but I remember that they'd wrap me in these hot pieces of wool. Then they'd put white towels over the wool, and finally they'd cover the whole works with plastic. The packs would be very hot when they put them on, and they were supposed to be changed while they were still warm. However, a lot of times they didn't get changed soon enough, and those "hot packs" became "cold packs!"

In addition to the heat treatment, I also had other therapy. I remember that a therapist used to come in and do passive exercises with my legs. She also would stretch me. We didn't have swimming or any other therapy though, at least not that I remember.

By some time in May, I guess the doctors felt that I had made enough progress to let me go home. I still had some paralysis in my left leg which resulted in my left foot being a "drop foot," and in order to walk, I had to sort of lock my knee. So when I went home, I had a small brace for that left foot. I went home on crutches, but before long, I threw those things away. I think that was just sort of the natural thing to do. As soon as I could get rid of something, I did!

I continued to wear the brace, but I didn't have any more therapy or exercises. I was an only child, and my mom and dad wanted to make sure that I got as much treatment as possible. So my parents talked to a friend of theirs who was a Shriner, and with his help, they were able to get me an appointment at the Shriners' Hospital, and we flew down there. I'm not sure of the exact date, but I know it was in November because the day before we left was election day. When I got up that morning, there were these wonderful political discussions going on. Harry Truman had just been elected president, and I remember asking, "Did we win?"

Truman's election was the only good thing that happened that day, at least as far as I was concerned. When we got to Shriners', the doctor examined me and said, "I think we'll keep her." I just burst out in tears and said, "You promised me I didn't have to stay here!" It wasn't that my parents had lied to me; they just didn't know if Shriners' could help me. But my parents explained to me it was for the best, so I was back in the hospital. I accepted it, but I sure wasn't happy about it. I figured I'd be in for another long stay, and I was. I was admitted in November, and I didn't get out until the next summer!

I was put in the "big-girls ward" and spent the first couple of weeks in an isolation cubicle. There were maybe five of those on that ward. I could see the rest of the girls, but a glass enclosure separated me from the others so that if I would have had chicken pox or some other contagious disease, it wouldn't be spread throughout the whole ward.

Things were very regimented on that ward. They got us up early in the morning; the beds were made, and we'd lie on top of these quilts that the Shriners' auxiliary had donated. The doctors made rounds on Monday, and your x-rays were laid out on a table. It was all very orderly. When the doctors came in your room, there was always a group of them including residents and interns, because they used that hospital as a teaching facility.

The first thing that they tried on me was "nerve stimulation." They put me under and pounded on my left leg with a rubber hammer or something. When I woke up that leg was all black and blue, and oh, did it hurt! They then wrapped the leg with hot packs, which reduced the pain a little. I guess they were trying to rejuvenate the nerves, but all it did was give me a sore leg!

Following that, a doctor came to examine me, and he looked at my brace and said, "We'll just throw this thing away. It's nothing but a mouse trap." And then he just took it and threw it in the closet across the room. I knew my parents had paid a lot of money for that brace, so I thought to myself, "It may be a mouse trap, but it's sure an expensive one!"

Not too long after they threw my "mouse trap" away, I had surgery on my left leg. I can still remember the name of the procedure. It was called a "triple arthrodesis." Though I still have a fence post for a left ankle, the doctors did everything they could to fix it up. They put in three staples to anchor the foot so it wouldn't have lateral movement, and they did a tendon transplant to give me up and down motion. After that surgery, I no longer had a drop foot, and I didn't need that "mouse trap" of a brace anymore.

Though I certainly didn't enjoy my hospital stay, I am very grateful to the Shriners. Not only did I get the best care possible, but they paid for almost everything. Based on what my initial hospitalization at St. Luke's cost, I'm sure that triple arthrodesis would have been very expensive. I know it took our whole wheat crop to pay the hospital bill from St. Luke's, and my dad said it had been his best wheat crop ever. Of course, back in those days, farmers didn't have medical insurance, so you just paid any doctor's bills in cash and hoped you didn't have any long hospital stays.

The March of Dimes didn't want to give us anything. They told my parents that there might be somebody else who needed help more. My mother was a feisty little dynamo, and she wouldn't take no for an answer. She found out that I was the only person in the whole county who had polio, so she went after the March of Dimes and finally did get some money from them, maybe $2,000, which helped a little.

It's a good thing that the Shriners paid my medical expenses, because I was back in the hospital again the next summer, which would have been 1949. At that time, my left leg was beginning to bow and become deformed, so they broke the long bone of the leg and reset it. They wanted to make sure that the leg healed correctly, so I was put in a cast that covered my hips and went all the way down the left leg. I spent several months in that cast. It was very uncomfortable, and when the incision started to heal, my leg really itched. They told me not to try and scratch it, but I did anyway. I got a knitting needle, and I'd reach down the cast very strategically and scratch as best I could. Thank God that I didn't get an infection.

When I finally got the cast taken off, the skin came off of that left leg, just like a snake skin! I needed a lot of physical therapy because I didn't have a full range of motion. I remember spending time in the whirlpool and then having the physical therapist try to stretch out that leg. She pushed and pulled so hard it felt like the leg was going to break again, but I guess that's what it took to get an adequate range of motion.

Though it sure wasn't any fun spending so much time in the hospital, it wasn't all bad. I remember that when the weather was nice, they would roll us outside onto the porch. That was the only chance we had to get outside, and we dearly loved it. Also, the Shriners did some special things for us. One year, Francis the Talking Mule came to the hospital to entertain us. And on your birthday or at Christmas, they would get you anything you wanted. It was always a big dilemma: what should I ask for? The only thing I really wanted though, was to go home. And I finally did go home, just in time to start the eighth grade.

I had missed a lot of school over the previous two years, but I did have tutoring, so I was able to keep up with my studies. I went to a small, country school, and it was quite a distance from our farm. Before I had polio, I used to go to school on horseback, but after my polio, I went by car. During the winter that I was in eighth grade, the weather was very bad, so I stayed with another family for about six weeks or so. Their farm was close to the school, and we went to school by horse drawn sleigh. That was fun.

I was really blessed to be with the kids at that school. They were just like family. There was no teasing. I know that some kids got teased a lot when they went back to school, but we were such a small group and had basically grown up together, so they just accepted me. I was included in everything. Of course, I wouldn't be chosen for some of the running games, but I did almost everything else. For instance, when we played softball, I would be the pitcher. I remember one time a boy hit the ball right back at me, and I couldn't get out of the way. The ball hit me right in the nose! But that didn't stop me from playing. Fitting in was important to me, and I did fit in pretty well.

I was also blessed to have such a good family. Everything was always positive at home. I do remember that my one aunt was always very concerned about how I looked, and she heard about this rubber stocking that could be put on over your leg to make it look "normal." Well, I took that to mean that if you don't look normal, then you are no longer the same person that you were. I know she was just trying to be helpful, but I resented that and spoke out about it, so that was the last I heard of it.

Anyway, the next year, I started high school. McHenry and Grace City were both small communities of less than 100 people, and I could have gone to high school in McHenry. However, Marlys, who was still my best friend, decided to go to high school in Grace City, so I decided to go there too. That way, I would not only be with my best friend, but we could ride to school together. That turned out to be a bad decision for me. The situation at Grace City High School was pretty bleak. It was such a small school that there were only two teachers there, and one of them was more interested in selling insurance than he was in teaching. They didn't seem to think that I had much potential, so there was no encouragement at all. And I didn't have the same social acceptance that I had in my elementary school. I remember going to the freshman dance. I was all excited about it, but no one asked me to dance all night! I was just crushed, and I remember thinking, "Is this the way things are going to be for the rest of my life?"

I wasn't one to complain or cry, but I think my parents sensed that things weren't going too well for me in Grace City. So the next summer we went to McHenry and talked to the principal of the McHenry High School about me transferring over there. He was very encouraging, and I remember him saying that he thought I would like it there. I didn't know any of the kids at McHenry High School, but I decided to give it a try, and it was the best move I ever made. I slowly made friends and started to get involved in a lot of school activities. I was in student council; I did some writing and eventually became editor of the school yearbook; and though I couldn't play on any sports teams, I sold tickets at the games. I even started to get asked to dances, and not just school dances, but community dances too. So, it was a really rewarding environment, and I never regretted transferring there. Believe it or not, when I graduated, I was the class valedictorian, or at least a "tri-valedictorian." We had eight or nine students in my graduating class, and three of us shared the distinction of being valedictorians!

Towards the end of my time in high school, I started to think seriously about what I was going to do after I graduated. I knew that I wanted to go to college, but I wasn't sure what I wanted to study. Ever since junior high, people had been telling me I should be a teacher, and I had thought about being a home economics teacher. I love to cook, but I can't sew worth a darn, so I didn't think I'd be too good at that. Then I started to think about occupational therapy. I knew I wanted to do something that involved working with people, and I really liked what the therapists did at Shriner's, so I thought, "Why not?"

Some people from the Division of Vocational Rehabilitation came out and met with my parents and me, and it was decided that I'd go to the University of North Dakota and study occupational therapy. The state would even pay for my tuition and books! So that's what I did, and I never regretted it. I did just about everything the other students did. I even took physical education classes. I learned to swim; I took a golf class; I even took dance. I joined a sorority, and I dated quite a bit, though never anything too serious.

It never crossed my mind that I couldn't do everything that I wanted to do. I even participated in the Foster County Dairy Princess Pageant. My mother had heard about it and signed me up. I ended up being the first runner-up. Actually, I should have won. I had more points than anyone else, but the judges said our dairy herd wasn't big enough, so my best friend Marlys's sister won. She was a beautiful girl, so I really didn't mind. In fact, I understood. They couldn't very well have a dairy princess with a leg that looked like a fence post representing Foster County in the state-wide pageant!

Getting back to my college experiences, I was a very good student, and in fact, some of my professors even suggested that I should change my major, perhaps to psychology, and go to graduate school for a masters or even a doctorate, but I really didn't want to do that. I wasn't really thinking about having a career. Back in those days, very few women could have a career and a family, and what I really wanted was to get married and have children. So I didn't want to go to graduate school. Instead, I wanted to be a homemaker.

I graduated with honors, but I didn't look for a job right away. Instead, I did some vacationing with my family and some friends, but my dad would tease me and say, "What are you going to do with that degree when the vacation is over. Don't you think you should look for a job?" I knew my dad was right, so after our vacation, I went down to the Veteran's Hospital in Fargo and interviewed for a job. As it turned out, they didn't have anything for me in Fargo, but there was a position in Des Moines, Iowa. I took the job, and it was wonderful. The director of the hospital was hearing impaired, and one of the women I worked with also had polio, so there was a good understanding of what it is like to be disabled. However, believe it or not, I never considered *myself* disabled, at least not back then.

I met my husband while I was working in Des Moines. He was a psychology intern there. After we were married, we moved to Tucson, Arizona where he finished his doctorate. We had four children, so I got my wish of being a mother and a homemaker. It's interesting, but some doctors had told me that I'd never be able to have children. Yet, I had no trouble with any of my pregnancies, and I had all normal, vaginal deliveries. Carrying the extra weight during my pregnancies was difficult, especially during the last two. That's when I started using crutches again. After my youngest was born, I realized that I needed to continue to use crutches even after I lost the weight I had gained during pregnancy. I didn't want him to get out of the stroller because when we'd go shopping or someplace that required a lot of walking, I'd use that stroller for a crutch.

Since then, it's just been a slow progression toward relying on the crutches more and more. My left knee is going, and I know I'll eventually need a knee replacement. I'm putting that off as long as I can though.

A doctor didn't tell me I needed to use the crutches. I guess I just prescribed them for myself. They take the weight off of my legs, especially my knees, and cosmetically, they don't bother me at all. Actually, I make a fashion statement with them. I have 10 or 12 pairs of crutches, and they're painted different colors to match my outfits. When my daughter got married in May, I had a jade green pair of crutches to match my jade green dress. My husband painted them for me. It was his idea, so that's been his contribution.

Anyway, after being a mother and homemaker for many years, I started working again in 1988. I am currently Coordinator of the Center for Independent Living here in Menomonie, Wisconsin, and my work involves training people to be peer advisors for others with disabilities. I'm also very involved politically in the handicapped rights movement. In fact, I'm a legislative coordinator, so I'm very much an advocate for people with disabilities.

When I stop and reflect on it, I can see the impact that polio has had on me and my life's journey. If I hadn't had polio, I doubt that I would have had the same professional aspirations that led me to my current career. Actually, I was very satisfied being on our farm and living in Foster County, but polio pushed me to broaden my horizons. So I very much think that having polio changed my life, and not necessarily all for the worse. I've thought this through because I do a lot of work with the grieving process, and if you'd say, "Well Mary Ann, you'll be able to run and dance and do all sorts of things that you've never been able to do," I'd say, "Yeah. That'd be great." But if I had to go back and not have the same life's journey, I think I'd say, "No thank you." It's been 45 years, and I like where I've gone and where I am. I don't like the disability, but I do like my life and the life's journey I've had.

Arvid Schwartz

I was born in 1940 on a farm near the town of Wood Lake in southwestern Minnesota. During the 1940's and early 1950's, farm life was quite different than it is today. Back in those days, we still did much of the farm work manually. We had a diversified farm with chickens, dairy cows, and pigs. We also raised crops. We had only one tractor, and we also farmed with horses. There were a lot of chores to do, and as the oldest son, I certainly did my share of them. We didn't have electric lights, at least not until 1946 when REA brought the line to our farm, and we had no running water, so we didn't have indoor plumbing. Conveniences were few and far between, yet my memories of life on our farm are very good ones.

In spite of all the work we did, we still had time for play. One of my favorite pastimes was riding my bike. I loved to ride my bike and still would love to ride one today if I could. However, in October of 1952, I had a bad fall, which was unlike me, because I was a very able bike rider. The day after my bike accident, I was carrying water to the hogs in a five gallon pail, and I was finding that difficult. In retrospect, I guess those were probably early signs that something was wrong, but at the time, I really didn't think anything of them.

A day or two later, I remember waking up and feeling quite ill. I was running a fever, and though I could still walk, I was stiff and sore. After a couple of days, my parents contacted the doctor. He came out and looked at me and told my parents that he thought I must have some kind of flu. However, though my parents did all the usual things that were done for flu back then, I continued to run a high fever. About three days after the doctor's visit, I vividly remember waking up in the morning and falling down when I tried to get out of bed.

My parents again called the doctor, and he came back out and looked at me. It was at that time that he brought up the possibility of polio, and he recommended that my parents bring me down to Sister Kenny Institute in Minneapolis. Now, at that time, my father had never driven to the Twin Cities in his life. He had no idea where the

Kenny Institute was, and only a vague notion that Minneapolis was somewhere east of Wood Lake! So he talked to his cousin who had been to the Twin Cities and tried to get some directions to the Kenny Institute.

I recall the day that I went down to the hospital very well. The date was October 21, and it was a beautiful day. Those on the neighboring farms were out in the fields picking corn. I clearly remember thinking to myself that I better take a good look around the farm because I might not be back there for a while. Unfortunately, that thought turned out to be prophetic.

My parents put me in the back seat of the car, propped me up, and we took off for the Twin Cities. Before we left, our doctor had made a call to Sister Kenny Institute and was told that they were full, and we should go to the University Hospital instead. So that's where we went, and I was admitted there about 5:00 P.M. I remember having the spinal tap, and then I was put in this stark little room. However, I didn't even spend one whole day at the University Hospital. About 10:00 P.M., they told my parents to take me over to Sister Kenny Institute, and I was admitted there. They took me up to the contagion ward, and I remember going down a hall filled with iron lungs and then into room 201.

Since I was in the contagion ward, my folks couldn't stay. Instead, they were sent over to the old Wisconsin Hotel, which was where Sister Kenny Institute sent parents who had brought children there. We couldn't see each other, and I've often wondered what sort of trauma they experienced. They had no idea what was happening to me, and the overworked doctors only knew me as one of the hundreds of polio patients at Sister Kenny, so they couldn't tell my parents much about my condition.

The situation must have also been very difficult for my brothers and sisters. They were all told that since they had been exposed to polio, they couldn't go to school for two weeks. My parents were in Minneapolis, and I believe that my grandmother came over to stay with them.

As far as my time in contagion, there were 10 or 12 of us in room 201. I think I spent seven or eight days there, and I can remember that time vividly. All I could do was lie there. I still had a fever, and my back was arched up into a half moon because my muscles had tightened up. They started using some hot packs on me, and I still have a scar on my abdomen from my first encounter with those hot packs. They were too hot when they put them on, and they burned me.

There was nothing for me to do, and I remember lying there and thinking about all the things I'd be doing if I wasn't in the hospital. I was just sort of mentally going through the day thinking, "Now I'd be going to this class; now I'd be home; now I'd be doing the chores." That's really all there was to do, other than stare at the ceiling and wonder what was going to happen next.

On the seventh or eighth day, they moved me out of the contagion room and put me in room 208, which was in the far southeast corner of the floor. Finally, my parents were allowed to see me, though they couldn't stay very long. We had a very brief visit, and I remember my father's lower lip was sticking out, quivering pretty badly, and I'd never seen that before. My mother was crying, and I'd hardly ever seen her do that. I didn't cry, but I remember telling them that I was probably going to need special shoes and that they'd be expensive, maybe as much as $18 or $20! I have no idea how I knew that, but our family stretched every dollar back then, and I was really concerned as to whether we could afford those "expensive" shoes. My dad just smiled and said, "Don't worry about that. We'll find the money to buy the shoes." Little did I know that I would also need braces that would cost 10 times more than the shoes!

Anyway, room 208 was a fairly large room that was probably supposed to accommodate six or eight beds. However, the hospital was so crowded that they had crammed about 14 beds into that room. I had no idea how long I was going to be there, though I had talked to some of the fellows who were in the room with me and learned that they had been there six or eight months. The thought of that long a stay was just daunting, but I think I was too young or too naive to know what was in store for me.

My early days in room 208 consisted basically of hot packs and then more hot packs. I dreaded them. They were hotter than hot, and before they would cool off, they'd come by and put on fresh ones. We had to lie on our backs with our feet up against the footboard. We weren't allowed to sit up or even lie on our stomachs, and we couldn't have a pillow. I remember that I would slide my hand under my back to see how arched it was. That was how I gauged my progress. I also knew I was making progress when I no longer needed catheterization and enemas!

Life in room 208 was pretty routine. Things were much the same, day after day after day. They woke us up in the morning, and after breakfast we had the first of our hot packs. There were two sessions of hot packs in the morning and one or two in the afternoon. I also remember that they did stretching with us. There was a great big guy who would come and do the stretching. It was quite painful, especially when he would stretch my leg muscles.

I must have made pretty good progress, because I was allowed to come home that Christmas on a three-day pass. I got out in the afternoon of Christmas Eve. I remember that when we got back to Wood Lake we drove into town to see the lights, and then we drove over to the church where the kid's Christmas program, in which I would have participated, was going on, and we parked outside. They were singing "Silent Night," and I remember rolling down the car window and listening. That was a very emotional experience for me.

Another thing that sticks out in my memory is that there were very few presents that Christmas, and one of the gifts to my brother was something I had made in the hospital. Here I had been concerned about my shoe costs, yet it had never dawned on me that there wouldn't be money for Christmas presents. We had no health insurance, and I'm sure the budget was very tight that year. As it turned out, the March of Dimes helped a lot with my polio expenses, but at that time, I'm sure my dad didn't have a clue regarding what the cost of my hospitalization would be or where that money would come from. He knew there were bills coming, and I'm sure he was saving any little bit he had to pay those bills.

As far as other memories of that Christmas, I know that I ate all the things that I wasn't supposed to eat. I got diarrhea, and of course, our outhouse wasn't handicapped accessible! When my parents brought me back to the hospital, they were worried that they were going to be reprimanded because of all the things they fed me. However, most of us came back in the same condition.

When I got back to the hospital, the treatment routine picked up right where it had left off. I believe that I had the hot packs until about February, and the end of those hot packs was another milestone and cause for celebration. After that, the therapy consisted mostly of stretching and reeducation of my muscles. Every day until I was discharged, they would take me into a little treatment room and stretch me and then lift and move my legs. I was supposed to push with my legs or straighten them after they had been bent, but my legs were pretty much completely paralyzed, so I couldn't do it. Muscles were rated by numbers, 1 through 10, and about once a week, they'd do those ratings. Unfortunately, I had a lot of zeros when they'd rate my legs. However, my back and arms were strong.

There was one day that we didn't get any treatment, and that was the day that Sister Kenny died. The head therapist came and announced that she had died and told us that if it wasn't for Elizabeth Kenny, the Institute wouldn't exist, and we wouldn't be getting the type of treatment that we were receiving. As a 12-year-old, of course, I really didn't grasp the significance of that.

Getting back to my treatment and therapy, every so often I had to go down to the clinic. Dr. Knapp would be there as would a bunch of other physicians. When they'd take you there, you'd be sort of put on display to demonstrate your situation or particular disability, and of course, we all hated that. I was always afraid of going there. I don't know if I was afraid that they'd find some new problem or if I was just scared of having to appear in front of all those doctors, but I sure know that I didn't like to go down there.

They had a "school" at Sister Kenny, and beginning probably sometime in February, I went to that "school" for about an hour and a half each day. We had an elderly lady for a teacher and a very strange classroom. There were three or four of us in our class, and we were all about the same age. I was in my wheelchair; there was a boy who was in a respirator, and a girl was wheeled down there in her bed. There may have been a fourth student, but I don't remember him or her. I went there for about three months. They sent a report card to my principal in Wood Lake. He looked at it and said I passed! So that's how I did my seventh grade.

Between our treatment and studies, there was time to have at least a little fun. One of the things we did in room 208 to entertain ourselves was to have spitball fights, and believe me; these weren't ordinary spitball fights. We somehow got a supply of rubber bands, and we'd tie two or three of them together and stretch them between our bedposts, which stuck up a little bit. After the lights were out, we'd use these giant slingshots to shoot spitballs at each other, and those spitballs would really fly. There were several beds on each side of the room and also two beds in the middle. Of course, those poor guys in the middle got bombarded from both sides. Eventually, we would make enough noise that the nurses would come down, and we'd catch hell. But really, what could they do to us?

The one thing that made my stay at Sister Kenny bearable was the fact that my parents never missed a visiting day. Visiting hours were from two to four on Sunday afternoon. It was a seven hour round trip, but my parents were there every Sunday with the exception of one time when they got caught in a snowstorm. I've thought about that over the years. Here was a man who had never driven to the Twin Cities, and now he was forced to go there every week. I really appreciate my mom and dad for that.

During those visits, my parents would fill me in on what was happening back home. They'd also bring me things. I remember that they used to bring me a packet of letters from my schoolmates back in Wood Lake, and they'd bring me books to read and maybe some candy or other good things to eat. Of course, candy was strictly forbidden, but other kid's parents would bring it, so I finally convinced mine to bring it as well. We'd hide the candy because periodically there'd be "raids," and our candy would be confiscated. We'd, of course, catch holy hell from the nurses, but we thought it was worth the risk. They even sent a letter home to our parents telling them not to bring us candy, and that worked for a couple of weeks, but then someone's parents would work up the courage to bring some, and the cycle would start over again until there'd be another raid.

At any rate, towards the end of May, I was transferred to Swedish Hospital in Minneapolis. Things were completely different at Swedish. Anything went over there. There was no lights-out rule, and we didn't have to go to therapy. You went only if you wanted. Visiting hours were unrestricted. In the evening, we'd go out in our wheelchairs and scoot around the block. I sometimes wonder if Swedish Hospital was purposefully set up that way to provide sort of a transition between Sister Kenny and life at home.

After three weeks at Swedish, I finally got to go home for good. They just came in and informed me I was being discharged. I really wasn't expecting it because no none had told me I'd be going home soon. But after I got the news, I just called my parents, and on June 19, 1953, they came and took me home.

So after eight months and two days in the hospital, I was finally back home. Being home was interesting. Before I left the hospital, I had been fitted with a long leg brace, and I was walking with Kenny sticks, or "kindling sticks," as we called them. Our house was certainly not set up for a person with a disability. For instance, all our bedrooms were upstairs, and we had one of those old farm stairways that curves around as you go up, and it had no handrail. So my dad bought a two-by-two, planed it down, and nailed it up. That's what I used to get up and down the stairs.

My dad was sure I would eventually be able to walk without the brace and the sticks, so he took an old water pipe and put the ends in the notches of two trees and made me walk between them as I held onto the pipe with one hand. I guess he thought that if I did that enough times, one day I'd just forget that I came to the end of the pipe and keep on walking without it. Of course, that never happened. I guess I knew early on that it wasn't going to work, but I sure don't blame my dad for trying.

I did go back to Sister Kenny Institute periodically for check ups, of course. I was always deathly afraid of going back there. I guess I was worried that they'd decide I needed surgery or something.

I never got any additional therapy at Sister Kenny, though. The only other therapy I got was from a chiropractor in Montevideo. My parents were believers in chiropractics, and they were sure this man could help me. So I went to see him for the better part of a year. For the first month, I lived with my uncle in Montevideo, and I went to the chiropractor twice a day for treatments. After that first month, I would go once a day, then three times a week, and so on. The chiropractor would photograph me and everything, because he thought he was going to cure me, and he wanted to have the photos to show my progress. Well, I'm not going to say that he didn't do me any good, but after that year, I still needed my brace and the Kenny sticks to walk. Eventually, I replaced those Kenny sticks with a pair of G.I. issue "sticks" when I was about 15. A fellow who had been injured in the military gave them to me, and I'm still using the same pair today. They just don't make them like that anymore. These babies were built to last!

At any rate, I returned to my one-room school in time to start the eighth grade. I had missed a whole year of school, yet I received no special help in readjusting. I just was put back into circulation like I had never been gone. I didn't get any special privileges and had all the same requirements as everyone else, and I think that was the right thing to do. I did have to stay in for lunch recess though, and my teacher, Mr. Grams, would stay in with me, and we'd play checkers or parchesi. We did that for that entire school year. I really appreciate the fact that he did that for me because I think it was a pretty big sacrifice for him. He was a young man in his late 20's, and he loved athletics, so I think he would have much rather been outside playing ball with the other kids.

After I graduated from the eighth grade, I went to the three-story public high school in town. I was kind of worried about that because I didn't know any of the teachers over there. Yet, I did fine. I got to and from my classes in two minutes just like everybody else, even if they were up two flights of stairs. The only concession the school made for me was that they made sure my classmates would carry my books between classes. I guess I was "mainstreamed" long before we knew what that word meant. Though I'm sure today there would be special ramps and handicapped accessible bathrooms, I have no regrets about doing it the hard way.

Actually, high school was a very positive experience for me. There were only about 80 kids in the entire school. They were all my friends and never seemed to notice that I was handicapped. The high school coach, who was kind of a rough, gruff guy, asked if I wanted to be the student manager for the sports teams. I thought that would give me a chance to be with my friends, so I did it. I ended up being sort of the score keeper and statistician for the football, baseball, and basketball teams. Another boy handled the equipment and did some of the other things that I couldn't do. I got to ride the team bus, and I went to all the games. I really liked that.

I was a good student in high school, and the other kids accepted me pretty well. The only thing that really bothered me was that I didn't date. I guess I figured that no one would want to go out with me, so I didn't have a girlfriend. I just thought it would always be that way, and I'd never get married.

After high school, I went to the Minnesota School of Business in Minneapolis. When I graduated, I took a job with the old St. Paul Fire and Marine, which is now the St. Paul Companies. I bought a car and had a blacksmith fit it with hand controls for me. Before I had the car, I used to ride the city buses, and back in those days, the buses weren't handicapped accessible, so getting on and off of them was quite a feat. I remember one time I was going out the back exit, and the bus driver closed the door and took off before I was completely out. My pants leg caught in the door, and I took quite a spill.

About the time I got my car, I also found a new friend. Actually, I think she found me! Judy, who's now my wife, was from my home town, but she was two years behind me in school, so I didn't know her very well. After she finished high school, she moved to the Twin Cities to work, and she didn't know anyone there. She gave me a call, and we started doing things together. At first, I didn't really consider it "dating," but we were together more and more, and I started thinking, "Wow, I've finally got a girlfriend." We got engaged in 1960, were married in September of 1961, and have had a wonderful marriage.

Back in those days, I guess I thought that "crippled" people didn't usually get married. Though I knew I would be a good husband and father, I had to convince one other person of that. Judy was and still is a beautiful woman who had been valedictorian of her high school class. I asked her to marry me realizing full well that friendship was one thing, but marriage was for life, and she might say no. We both realized that my handicap would require her to do some extra things that I just couldn't do. It's impossible to describe the joy I felt when she said yes. She told me that she had indeed thought about the "complications" that might result from my handicap, but she knew that together, we could work through them. And we have worked through them, not only to have a wonderful marriage, but to still be best friends.

We have two terrific children, Lance and Carolee. Both are married and launched in their careers. Having children posed some special, and sometimes humorous, problems. Yet we always figured out a way to get things accomplished. Our kids have never complained about the fact that their dad has a handicap. In fact, I think they are proud of the way we've worked things out in spite of it.

Anyway, I stayed at St. Paul Fire and Marine for only about eight months, and then I went to work for a C.P.A. firm as a junior auditor. One of their clients was a company called Group Health Plan, which was a pre-paid medical care organization, and sort of a forerunner of the H.M.O. One day a week, I did the books for them. As that company grew, I started spending more of my time there, and eventually, I went to work for them. I started in 1961 and worked my way up until I eventually became the treasurer and financial vice president. While I was employed there, I took evening courses at Metropolitan State University, and completed my college degree. In 1985, the president of the company, with whom I had worked for 25 years, retired. With his retirement and the "changing of the guard" there, I chose to leave the company about a year later.

I had no idea what I was going to do. I guess I was experiencing somewhat of a mid-life crisis. After all, I had two kids in college; we were building a new home, and I didn't have a job! However, by that time, a friend and I were involved in land development in the Twin Cities as kind of a hobby. That proved to be a very successful enterprise, so I started to spend more time on that. I was also becoming very involved on a national level with the Wisconsin Synod

Lutheran Church, which took a lot of my time.

Though I hadn't done farm work since my youth, farming had always been in the back of my mind. I was still a farmboy at heart, and so when the opportunity came along to trade some lots for farm land, we decided to do it. I didn't intend to farm it myself. Rather, I figured that I'd rent it to someone else. We found a young couple who wanted to get started in farming, but rather than renting the land to them, we formed a farming partnership instead.

I started coming out to the farm pretty regularly, and eventually, my wife said to me, "As long as you're out there so much, why don't we just move there?" So in 1989, we built a home on our land and moved down here. Our farm has grown to 2000 acres, and we have a fairly large livestock operation. Though it was never my intention to actually do my own farming, I eventually figured out how to get on one of the tractors, and that was so exhilarating there was just no stopping me. I found that I still loved farming, and I started doing more and more. I don't do the planting, because I can't handle the seed bags, and I don't work with chemicals. However, I do the field preparation; I cultivate, combine, bale hay, and everything else.

I did find it difficult to get into a lot of the equipment though, so I went to a local blacksmith and had him modify some of it for me. When I bought a new combine, I went to Indiana and talked to a man who works with the Breaking New Ground Program at Purdue University. He put an electric lift on the combine, and I now can easily get into it.

So things have turned out well for me. I'm enjoying my return to farming. I'm still involved in my other business interests, and I'm very active with our church, both locally and on a national level. I sing in our church choir, and I'm a member of the Board of Trustees for the Wisconsin Evangelical Lutheran Synod. I also serve on the Board of Regents for Wisconsin Lutheran College, which is in Milwaukee, and I'm on the Board of St. Croix Lutheran High School in St. Paul.

I feel that I've been very fortunate in many ways. In spite of polio, I have had a very successful career and a wonderful family life. Though I'm now wearing braces on both legs, I still get around quite well with my G.I. issue "sticks." I don't believe that I've had any post-polio symptoms, which is a good thing. As you can see, I'm just too busy for that!

As far as putting some closure on this, I'd just like to share two thoughts that have been with me since I had polio. The first is that life is like a deck of cards. You get dealt a hand, and you only have two choices. You can throw them in or play them. My choice has always been to play them. With God's help, I think I've played my hand pretty well.

Secondly, as a Christian, I know that God's plans for me are far better than my plans for myself. Though some days I still long to be able to run and ride my bike, I know that a lot of other good things have happened to me because of the fact that I've had polio. It's a waste of valuable time to try and figure it all out, so I simply say to myself, "To God be the glory!"

Diane Keyser

I had polio when I was 12, and I distinctly remember the day that I was diagnosed. It was Saturday, September 10, 1949. I started getting sick the day before. I had a tingling feeling in the skin of my stomach and legs, and I felt very sick to my stomach. I remember my mother giving me grape soda and making custard for me, and it took many years before I could stand the sight of either of those foods again. I believe it was on that same day we called the doctor, and he came up to the house. After examining me, he sent me to the hospital by ambulance.

I got to the hospital and went directly to the children's ward. I distinctly remember them doing the spinal puncture. I had to lie on my side, and they drew my knees up to my chest. I had severe pain while they did that. I can still remember it like it happened yesterday. Then they took me back to my room. I remember getting out of bed and looking up and down the hall. I believe that was the last time I walked on my normal legs.

My stay in the hospital was almost four months. The first couple of weeks I was flat on my back, and I had bad pain every time they turned me over on my side. I couldn't turn over by myself. I was put in an isolation ward, and I remember my mother and father standing by the door talking to me. They couldn't come in the room, however. I don't think that I had a lot of pain except when I put one leg on top of the other, so I just kind of laid there. It was a very hard time. I remember that I asked my dad if he could bring me a "Coney dog."

After I was out of isolation, they started putting hot packs on me. They did that every couple of hours. They used very hot blankets that they had put in some kind of water. They also started stretching my legs and back and arms.

I can also very vividly remember an incident that occurred in the hospital. They put me in a bathtub in a small room. I don't know if they forgot about me for a while, but I remember the water was dripping out of the tub, and I couldn't reach the faucet to turn it off. I also remember the many nights that I couldn't sleep at all, so the hospital stay seemed like an eternity. We listened to the radio in those days, and I remember listening to "The Shadow." That seemed to help pass the time.

It was a big thing that I had polio, and I received many gifts and cards. I believe that I almost died, so everyone was praying for me at our church. My brothers and sisters couldn't live at home with my parents because it was thought that they might also get polio. They had to stay in different places during the period that I was in isolation.

After being in the hospital for about four months, I came home in a wheelchair because I was still unable to walk. Then my parents took me down to Milwaukee to get a leg brace. I started walking a little bit with the help of that brace and some crutches.

We lived in Manitowoc, Wisconsin, and they didn't have any physical therapy or orthopedic services for me there at that time, so I was sent away to Sheboygan, Wisconsin. I lived in a foster home during the week and attended the orthopedic school where they had a physical therapist. I got physical therapy every day. They put me in a hot tub, and I had stretching and exercises. The physical therapist basically taught me how to walk again.

I was there for about nine months, and it was a very sad period of my life because I was a seventh grader, and I was missing out on what normal kids do during adolescence. I remember that they had a school bus that would take me back to the foster home after school, and I would just sit there alone all night and listen to the radio. There was no TV back in those days, of course.

I did get to come home on weekends, but my friends were all busy already, going here and going there. I couldn't keep up with them anyway. I remember it as being a very, very painful year for me. I was wearing a right leg brace at the time, and I needed crutches to walk. I think I wore the leg brace for almost a year. Then it broke. We sent it away to get repaired, but by the time we got it back, I had learned how to walk without it. I would push my knee way back. I had to do that because I had no muscle control in my right knee.

With or without a brace, it was always very hard for me to walk on ice. My parents wanted me to be independent, and the doctors encouraged them to allow me to do things on my own. However, I remember one time walking home from high school, which was only three blocks from my house, and I fell down on an icy road and couldn't get up. I laid there for quite a while before someone saw me, helped me up, and brought me home. I had many, many bad falls on the ice. One time when I was still using crutches and wearing the brace, I swirled around on the ice and landed flat on my back. I guess that's why to this day I dread ice. I'm more careful now, and as a result I don't fall as often as I used to.

What other impact did polio have on my life? Well, I guess the hardest part was being a teenager and trying to keep up with my friends. I loved sports, particularly basketball, but I couldn't play it. The only thing I could do was swim. During school when all the kids were in sports, I would have to sit on the side and watch.

Another thing that I particularly remember is I'd go with my friends to polka dances, and I couldn't dance. That really bothered me a lot, because I really would have loved to dance. I guess that I think having polio is hardest when you're a teenager.

As far as the impact of polio on my adult life, I'm fortunate that I have a husband and three beautiful children. I have a nice home, and a good job as a cytologist, which involves examining pap smears. In the past, I have done this work right at my home, so I didn't have to go out during the winter and worry about the ice. However, I now use my wheelchair and work 32 hours a week at a clinic.

For many years, I was able to walk without the use of braces, crutches, or a wheelchair. In fact, I could walk so well that I almost ended up being a registered nurse. Then I fell down on the ice and hurt myself, so I never continued in that. Instead I got into cytology and have had a very good career.

Though I thought that I would never need braces or crutches again, by the time I was in my 40's, my bad knee began to deteriorate and really started hurting. When I was 53, I had to start wearing a leg brace again.

I remember going down to the clinic in Marshfield, Wisconsin to get the brace fitted, and they put the leg brace on me. Then they put these shoes on me, and they were so ugly. As they were putting this stuff on, the tears just came out of my eyes. I thought, "I'll never get used to this. I can't even take a step." It felt like such a step backwards after going all those years without needing a brace.

Although I took the brace home, I just let it lay around for a couple years. I simply couldn't bring myself to wear it. However, my leg started hurting more and more, and finally I gave in and decided I would just have to get used to wearing a brace again. At first it took me almost half an hour just to put it on, but now I'm very used to it. It's like I've erased it from my mind. However, it still makes my foot feel like it's bound. It hurts in different areas if I wear it too long, so I try to take it out of my mind completely.

Though readjusting to wearing a brace was difficult, I guess the hardest part in my adult life was before I started using my wheelchair. I always would worry about going to weddings or other functions. Could I get in this place? Were there steps? Would I be able to get around without slipping on the ice or the dance floor? Could I get through the crowds without falling? It's such a pressure on a person's brain. It's hard to explain to someone who hasn't experienced it.

Do I think my life would have been different if I wouldn't have had polio? Yes, I think it would have been very different; I believe that my life would have been much more enjoyable because I would be able to take walks, run, ride horses, dance, and not have to worry about falling or whether I could get into or out of a place. I would be able to wear high heels instead of having to wear a brace and flat shoes.

I'm really not feeling sorry for myself though. I realize that I have many, many good things in my life. I have a lot of things that other people don't necessarily have. A lot of people who didn't have polio have probably had a more difficult life than I've had.

I've always been determined to get through this. I decided that if I was going to feel sorry for myself, I was the only one who would suffer. I've always had the attitude that I have to conquer this thing and go on living, and I think I have. I think I'm almost always a positive thinker, and I don't believe that I ever really let polio get me down.

Over the last couple of years, I believe that I've started to feel some effects of post-polio syndrome. I've been relying on my wheelchair more, and I tire a lot more easily that I did, but I'm not going to allow myself to worry about it. Rather, I intend to just go on with my life. What else can I do?

Chapter 7

Adult Polio

Polio has always been thought of as a disease that primarily affected children. In fact, it was called "infantile paralysis" in the first third of the 20th century. However, as demonstrated by the relatively large number of Allied soldiers who contracted polio during World War II, adults were certainly not immune to the disease.

Of those we interviewed for this project, only the three women whose stories appear in this chapter developed polio as adults. Two were pregnant at the time. All three women recovered relatively well from their initial bouts with polio. However, two currently are experiencing what would appear to be post-polio related difficulties, and the third, Evelyn Finks, later developed multiple sclerosis (MS). Though Evelyn speculates that there may be a connection between polio and MS, there is no research to substantiate such a connection. Rather, polio was and MS is a relatively common disease. Therefore, some individuals are likely to contract both. Evelyn Finks has the misfortune of being one of them.

June Radosovich

In August of 1952, I was 23 years old and working at the Deerwood Bank in Deerwood, Minnesota. At that time, I was a really active person. I played golf a lot; I swam a lot; I worked. I was dating. You know, busy, busy all the time. Somehow I contracted a cold. However, I still kept doing all of the fun things that I liked to do, and I still went to work. I was a big movie buff and went to every change of movies back then. We only lived two blocks from the theater, and one night I thought I was getting over the cold, so I washed my hair and said, "Mom, I'm going to the movies." My mom said that maybe I better not because I was just beginning to feel better, but I told her I was feeling really good, and so I went to the movie even though I still had a little bit of a damp head. The next day I came home from work, and I wasn't feeling well at all. That's how it all started.

I remember feeling really tired for the next several days. I think I was home for about a week before I went to the hospital. It got so I couldn't keep anything in my stomach, and each day I could feel my body getting weaker; it felt kind of like jelly. I would sit up in bed or push myself up in bed, and I would just slide right back down. We called the doctor, and my sister said to him, "I think she has polio." That was the year, 1952, when everybody was getting the symptoms and worrying about it because there was such a big epidemic. The doctor told her, "No, I don't think she has it," but he said that I should go to the hospital and get a spinal tap to make sure. Sure enough, they found out that I had polio. It was so bad by then that they called a priest right away, and I was in the ambulance and on my way to Sister Kenny Institute that very same day.

I remember riding in the ambulance, and I remember some of the things about getting there and how they put me on the cart and lifted my leg and my knee up and how my legs would go right back down. They would not stay in a bent position. Then they put me in a room. My mother and my sister had to leave, but I remember being in the room with another young girl. The room was kind of dark, or at least that's how it seemed to me, and I was drifting in and out of consciousness. About the only other thing I recall is that the doctor came in and said to the other girl, "Don't complain; we're busy fighting for this other gal's life over here." I remember that. I knew that "other gal" was me, so I knew that I wasn't doing too well!

I spent the next three months at Sister Kenny Institute, and I remember it as being a wonderful place with wonderful doctors. We were stacked up like cord wood there because so many people, particularly children, had polio that year. Kids were lined up side by side. Yet, they still managed to give us the very best care possible.

I remember that the doctors were all really interested in how I might have contracted polio. They probably still don't know how it's transmitted to this day. Well, maybe they know now, but they sure didn't know then how you caught it. I know that I had counted the pennies of a little girl who had died from polio. They brought her piggybank over to the Deerwood Bank, and I counted her pennies, so maybe I caught it from her somehow. Who knows?

But at Sister Kenny, they wanted to know everything I could possibly think of concerning how I might have gotten it. I was in a run down condition, they think, because I had been sick with a cold and my resistance was lowered, but they still didn't know how I actually got it.

Deerwood is a small town, and as far as I know, there was just that one little girl who had it that year. I don't know if it came from contact with germs on her pennies or not. It's weird that you don't know how or why you were singled out.

Anyway, at Sister Kenny, they eventually put me upstairs with all of these other polio patients, and I couldn't have any visitors. Every day I was there, and I don't know how long it was, but every day, I got more paralyzed. I could feel the pain go from my right arm to the shoulder, then to my neck, and then to the left arm. By that time, I couldn't move anything but my left hand. I had what they called "Bulbar polio" which affected my lungs. I couldn't see part of the time, and I couldn't go to the bathroom. They tried to put me in an iron lung, but I remember fighting that. I didn't want to go in there. I'm sure that if I couldn't breathe at all on my own they would have just done it. But because I fought going into the iron lung, instead, they put me in an oxygen tent.

I don't remember how long I was in that, but all the while I had a high fever, and I was really sick and in pain. Once the fever broke, the pain started to go away, and the paralysis quit spreading, but by that time I had it all over anyway. I basically had it everywhere. Thank goodness most of it didn't last.

After the fever left, they started treatment, and little by little by little, the paralysis started leaving. I've been left with a lot of residuals that you can't always see, but nothing really obvious. However, it took a long time and a lot of treatment before they could get me out of bed to try to walk or do anything else.

I remember that we had a regular daily treatment routine at Sister Kenny. First of all, I couldn't get out of bed, so they had a board at the end of the bed, and they stretched you out, putting your feet against the board, so you would never curl up. That's the way we had to sleep all the time. Then, all day long for six to eight hours a day, they gave us the treatment with hot packs. There were full packs and partial packs. They took boiling hot rags out of something that looked like a washing machine. Your body had to be completely dry before they put them on you, or you would be burned. They put these hot towels all over your body and then left you covered with plastic to keep the heat in. They would leave you in these hot packs from head to toe for a half an hour. Then they alternated with partial packs which they would just lay on you, and you could turn on your side. Those stayed on for an hour at a time. Like I said, this went on for six or eight hours a day.

They started the hot packs right after I got out of the contagion ward, and it continued all the while I was there. I wasn't able to eat; I hadn't eaten for weeks on end. I remember that they'd do everything to try to get you to eat. They also tried anything to get you to go to the bathroom. They'd turn the faucet on; they'd pour water on your tummy; they'd make you gurgle with water into a straw, anything to make you go the bathroom, and anything to make you get something wet in your mouth. It took them three hours to give me four teaspoons of water the first time I ate anything. When you haven't eaten for weeks on end, it's so hard to eat.

I know that they did give me something intravenously though, at least when I was in the oxygen tent. I remember that because a couple of times the needle came out, and the fluid went into my arm. That was very painful.

It took a long time before I could have a bath, and I had to be put into the tub and wait for somebody to come and drag me out. One time my girlfriend came and washed my hair. That was great! Eventually though, I got to the point where they could get me out of bed, stand me up, and I could walk into the bathroom. By that time I was able to go to the bathroom by myself, but it took a long time before any of my reflexes worked. I lost my regular swallowing mechanism, but somehow I developed a second set of reflexes that help me swallow.

After they got me up, I started getting a little better, and they started to reeducate my muscles. They did that by just bending the fingers, or bending the wrist. None of my muscles worked, so that's how they began my therapy. As I got a little stronger, they started the "hurting" method of therapy which really did hurt just as much as being sick. They would take my torso and just twist it or bring my head down and move my arms. It really hurt! My bones and muscles were whacked out of shape. The pain was as if you've injured your back, and it's stiff and sore, and then someone comes and pounds you or turns you. That's really how it felt. I always used to say it was just as painful to get well as it was to get sick because it hurt so much!

Because of all the patients they had at Sister Kenny, they eventually transferred me over to Mt. Sinai Hospital after my condition was stabilized. I think I was at Mt. Sinai for maybe three weeks. I got home from there out of sheer determination. I had to walk part way down the hall and show them that I could do a few other things before they'd let me go home.

After I was released from the hospital, they gave me exercises that I had to do at home and that my family had to do with me. We did that every day to try and reeducate the muscles. It hurt, but gradually as I got better and stronger, it didn't hurt as much. The family support was great. That helped a lot. Other people from my hometown were just wonderful to me too. When I came back, they wrote articles in the paper, and everyone tried to help me with things. They came to see me and took me out. They were just great, the whole town.

I spent about a year using Australian sticks, which were like wooden and leather crutches, but I got stronger all the time. I had so much help from my family in doing the exercises and everything that I was able to get rid of those crutches relatively quickly.

I had to go back to the hospital every week to be checked, and I went back to Sister Kenny and another hospital for several years, until I finally realized nothing else was going to get any better. I wasn't left with any permanent paralysis, but there are things I can't do, things that you can't see. Quite a few parts of my body are not strong, and those muscles just never completely recuperated.

I believe all of the treatment I received worked. I really do, but never the less, I was left with scoliosis of the spine, and after all these years, my rib cage is twisted. My rib cage on the right is kind of bowed. I have very weak stomach muscles. In fact, I had to wear braces because I have such weak trunk muscles, and I had nothing to hold me up. I was just floppy. I wore the body brace for maybe seven or eight years. It was very uncomfortable. There were metal stays in the back and front, and straps around my arms and legs, but I had to have it until I got strong enough to be able to maneuver myself. Eventually though, I got to the point where I did well without the braces, so I stopped wearing them. I still had to wear sturdy shoes with a lift in them for walking, but I never needed any braces for my legs.

When I would go back down to Sister Kenny, I went through the whole rigmarole of x-rays and examinations. In fact, I worry about that. I worry about being exposed to so much radiation, because the x-rays in those days weren't as good as they are now, and they gave me lots of x-rays. However, nothing has happened yet, and it was good treatment back then.

I was really very fortunate considering all the impairment I initially had that I ended up in such good shape. I'll tell you one thing though; you have to help yourself. You have to be determined, and that's just the type of person I am. I made up my mind I was going to get well. I knew that I'd have to do it on my own, and I did.

Of course, the doctors helped! I remember the doctor I would see at Sister Kenny for my check-ups. Because I had so much involvement, they put me in the hands of Doctor Miland Knapp. He's a world renowned doctor. He's written and traveled in Europe, all over. He ended up being my outpatient doctor.

As far as my life after having polio, of course I couldn't do a lot of the things that I used to do. I missed them, but it's funny; I really didn't think that I had things taken away from me until I got older. In the last 10 years or so, I realized I missed a lot of things I used to love to do. I guess it never bothered me then because I was just concerned about getting well.

Something that's really strange though, is that two of my girlfriends developed polio a few years after I had it, maybe in 1955 or 1956. One of the girls is dead now, but I remember that her mother came to me and asked me where I had been and what kind of treatment I had undergone; their family had a lot of money. I stressed that she should go to Sister Kenny because they try to make you help yourself. They really impressed that on you, that you've got to help yourself. She went there, but it wasn't a big beautiful hospital where everybody waits on you. Patients were there to get well, to help themselves, and so her mother took her out of there and put her in a hospital that was more luxurious. That wasn't the right thing to do, and she just didn't get as well as she could have.

We weren't even together at that time, so I don't think she could've caught it from me. It makes me think that maybe when we were younger we got the bug and that it takes certain circumstances to bring it out; I don't know. I probably will never know.

As far as my current life, I'm married and have two grown sons, both of whom were born by Cesarian section. I had no trouble with my pregnancies, as far as carrying the children, even though that was extra weight on my back. Actually, I felt really physically great when I was pregnant.

My husband and I have been married for 39 years, and he's an angel to me. He always has been. He does a lot of the heavy things for me now. In the beginning, I could do everything, or at least I found a way to do everything. I was determined to do anything I wanted, and I pretty much did.

I'm slowing down some now, and I'm having a little bit of difficulty. I can't get up stairs very easily. If I carry something, forget it. Then I can't get up the stairs at all! If I carry something in my left arm, even just the mail from work, I have difficulty just walking, even when I'm not going up stairs. I tend to lose my balance, and I don't have the stamina that I used to have. I'm older, too, and that makes a big difference, and I just can't do as much as I used to.

I don't think it's just because of my age though. I can tell what is from age and what is from the polio. Sometimes I wonder if I have some of that post-polio syndrome that I've heard about. When I'm out in the kitchen cooking, all of a sudden I realize I just can't stand there any longer. I find myself slumping over. It's the upper torso that's causing it. I love to cook, and on the weekends I do just fine, but during the week, I get very tired. I end up getting things done out of sheer determination. However, sometimes I just can't do something, and I have to quit and sit down.

For a while I was even going to go back to the doctor and see if I had post-polio syndrome because I was so tired, but I'm feeling better lately. Maybe it was just some quirk. I guess if I really thought I had post-polio syndrome, I would go back and try and find Dr. Knapp. But as it is now, I just go to our clinic here.

I have, of course, thought from time to time about what my life would have been like if I hadn't had polio, wondering what more I could have done, where I might have been. Maybe I would have moved to another state. Although I did that too. I lived in California for a while. Maybe I would have gotten into something more athletic. I don't know that I would have, but I might have, because I was an active, outdoors person.

I've been happy with my life, however, and I haven't suffered that much throughout the years. It could have been a lot worse. I get frustrated sometimes because I can't do all of the things I want to do; that's the biggest thing. Yet, I don't ever dwell on it. Rather, I'm just grateful that I'm still functioning reasonably well. I'm enjoying my grandkids and taking life one day at a time.

Evelyn Fink

I am Evelyn Fink, and I guess you would consider me a survivor of the polio epidemic of 1953. I was married in December of 1952, and my husband and I moved to Indianapolis, Indiana right after our wedding. I had quit my teaching job at St. Mary's College in Notre Dame, Indiana to move down there to live with my husband. I got pregnant in April, and during the first trimester of my pregnancy I caught polio.

My husband and I had gone to a swimming pool at the Riviera Club in Indianapolis with a family that had three boys. That occurred on a busy Saturday. The next day the mother of the boys called. She told me that her three-year-old son had not been able to get out of bed that morning, and the doctor had diagnosed him as having polio.

I went to the doctor and got gamma globulin shots. There was no polio vaccine yet, so gamma globulin shots were all they could give you to try to prevent you from getting polio.

A week after having gone to the pool with that family, I developed the typical symptoms of polio. I had a temperature, an aching back, and a headache as I lay in bed for three days. My obstetrician was on vacation, so I called a general practitioner who had been recommended to me. He prescribed an antibiotic which didn't do any good. All it did was make me sicker than I had been at any time during my pregnancy.

In addition to the headache and neck pains, I started to feel like I had a charley horse in my right calf. I mentioned this to the doctor, and he said, "Well, we could always put you in a camp corset."

I kept complaining about this intense pain. The thing that I had that was kind of different was I had a pain in my chest from about two to four in the morning. It was so excruciating that I would move out to the sofa bed in the living room because I couldn't stand it without feeling like I was going to scream. The doctor gave me phenobarbital to help me sleep.

I then became very depressed. I suppose it was because I was a new bride who had given up my teaching position to move to Indianapolis with my husband, and now, all of a sudden, the whole enormity of being really sick for the first time in my life hit me very hard. I didn't have a car and couldn't even get out at all. I became terrified of my own thoughts and had my husband take my phenobarbital pills with him to work every day.

It wasn't until October, about three months after I first got sick, that my obstetrician finally sent me to an orthopedic specialist in Indianapolis. He told me that I had polio and that it had affected the achilles tendon in my right leg. He gave me a muscle relaxant medicine and told me to have my husband wrap my leg in hot, wet towels. My husband Russ would spread a plastic table cloth on the bed and then bring steaming hot towels and wrap them around my legs. Then he'd fold the table cloth over me. I think that was the Sister Kenny method of trying to relax the muscles as much as possible.

It was not until our son was born on the 15th of January that I had any idea about the worries that my doctor had about me delivering a healthy baby. It seems they were expecting me to give birth to a monster. Today, I suppose they would recommend an abortion, but back in those days, they didn't think so much in terms of abortion. Thank goodness for that, because I had a normal, terrific son and named him Michael.

We moved back to South Bend in January, 1955. It was then that the Salk vaccine came out. Our son had the vaccine, and after our daughter was born, she was also vaccinated.

After I recovered from the polio, I didn't notice anything particularly different about my walk except that I could no longer skip or hop or dance because I had a paralyzing feeling in my right foot and ankle. We lived in a Cape Cod home at that time, and it had 13 steps up to the house, and then stairs down to the basement. I was still able to go up and down the stairs without a problem. It wasn't until 1961 that we needed to build a ranch style home so that I wouldn't have to go up and down stairs.

It was also in 1961 that I went back to teaching. However, I soon started to develop what was later diagnosed as multiple sclerosis (MS). I was initially hospitalized with what my neurologist called Guillain-Barre Syndrome and was left with residual feelings of tingling and weakness. At the time, I did not realize that this was the beginnings of MS.

It wasn't until 1984 that I finally learned I had MS. I had gone to the doctor because I had heard about post-polio syndrome. After having a battery of tests, I was diagnosed with MS rather than post-polio syndrome. Actually, if the beginning of my MS was in 1961, that would have been quite a long period of remission. My reason for bringing this up is that I truly believe there are enough polio survivors who now have MS that I can't help but wonder if there is some connection between the two.

Jeanne Molloy

In August of 1954, I was 22 years old and about seven months pregnant. My husband was in the Army, and we were living at an Army base in Kentucky where we shared an apartment with another Army couple. The last thing in the world I expected was to get polio, but yet, that's what happened.

I remember very vividly standing up one morning and feeling like I had the flu. I just collapsed. My husband had to report for duty at seven or eight o'clock, so he had to leave, but he placed a call to get me some assistance. An Army social worker came over to our apartment, and she decided I should be taken to the hospital right away. The other couple's husband had to carry me because by that time I was so weak that I couldn't walk from the car to the hospital. My legs just wouldn't support me anymore. It wasn't painful or anything. I would just get up and collapse.

When I got to the hospital, they took a spinal tap right away, and they came in very quickly afterwards and asked, "Do you think that you have polio?" I didn't think that I did because I didn't believe anybody my age could get it, but that's what I had!

The rest of that day is kind of a blur. I was put in isolation, of course, and they immediately took my husband out of circulation and put him in isolation for a while too. Thank God that he didn't get it, so they let him out of isolation in just a few days.

My parents had been down to visit us just that weekend, and I was very concerned about them. They were not put in isolation because they had returned home by that time, and fortunately, neither of them came down with polio. I was their only child though, and it was very hard on my parents because there wasn't a thing they could do for me. We were in the Army, so I was cared for. But they couldn't see me very often because of the distance factor.

I can remember as a child growing up and being kept away from crowded places because my parents were afraid that I'd get polio, which was so rampant in the forties and early fifties. Then I became an adult and got it! It was kind of an ironic twist of fate.

In addition to being difficult on my parents, I think my polio was kind of a test for my marriage. My husband stood by me, though. We had only been married for two years, and my illness actually proved to be a great bonding experience for us. So maybe some good came out of it.

The doctors seemed to think I was very contagious, but I have my doubts about that. Maybe some types of polio might have been contagious, but I don't think that mine was. If it was, I would think that my husband or the couple we were living with would have gotten it, but I was the only one who did.

My stay at the hospital was very long, about five months, from that August, 1954 until February, 1955. I remember getting the treatment with the hot packs where they'd wrap your limbs and just sort of let you simmer for a while. Believe me, on a hot, August night in Kentucky, the last thing in the world you want is a hot pack!

I ended up having my baby late. I was due in October, and Glenn wasn't born until November first. He was perfectly healthy; my polio didn't affect him at all. However, because of the pregnancy, I couldn't get up and start walking again right away. I did have some physical therapy, but it was limited. So, it was only after Glenn was born that I was able to go into more intensive physical therapy and start walking again.

I remember being in a ward with two other women. We had quite a comradery between us. They had been pregnant, and both had lost their babies. Fortunately, I was much further along than they were. They were in the early stages of pregnancy. However, I was still concerned about the polio affecting my baby, though the doctors didn't seem all that concerned. Of course, the Army is a very impersonal mechanism. They didn't seem too concerned about anything. I remember my husband asking, "Well, when do you think she'll be released from here? Maybe by Christmas?" And one of those Army doctors who had no more desire to be there than we did just looked at him and said, "What year?"

I did have a positive experience when the baby was born. Dr. McLaverty, who was very Irish, had a wife who had been in the hospital at the same time as me, and I chatted with her and told her I had seen her husband, and he was such a kind soul. I very much wanted to have him deliver my baby. I thought there was no chance for that to happen, but yet he made special arrangements for when I delivered, and he was there after all. So some individuals were very warm and caring.

Fortunately, the physical therapists who worked with me were very good. I remember one very vividly, a Lt. McKinley. She was very encouraging. The therapy was painful at first, because I was stretching the muscles that had been shrunk. But she just had a marvelous sense of humor, and that sort of got me through it. She used to bring me the *New Yorker* to read and things like that. She had to come and stretch those muscles, and I would want to pull the sheets up over my head and hide, but working with her made it bearable.

They kept testing me for my percentage of muscle loss. They didn't seem to think my muscle loss was too severe, but when I started to stand up again and walk, I wondered if they were right. I remember quite vividly that learning to walk again was a very difficult process. Yet, they got me back up and going pretty quickly. I guess I'm just that sort of person. I always thought, "I am going to walk again." There was never any question in my mind that I wouldn't be able to walk. I was going to walk again; I just knew it.

I wore a hip brace, and I remember being terrified of standing at the top of stairs with crutches and that brace because I thought I might fall. There were people right there with me, but I couldn't even get myself to try coming down stairs. It was terrifying. However, the fear gradually subsided. I still have a very weak sense of balance though, and I brace myself, at least a little. If I stub my toe, I'll try to prevent myself from falling because I used to fall quite often. Stairs are still hard for me. I have to take them one at a time when I'm going up.

After I finally got out of the hospital, I went back on almost a daily basis for therapy which was a little difficult to manage with a new baby. My husband Don had to carry me in and out. I had a wheelchair, but it was easier for him to carry me into most places because nothing was wheelchair accessible back then. That went on for several months until about June or so. After that, I didn't seem to have many more checkups. They seemed to think I had improved about as much as I could.

I could feel myself getting stronger all the time. First I got rid of the crutches. Then I started feeling more confident about walking and knowing I could make it from here to there without falling. They told me that I might walk better if I had surgery, but I seemed to be doing just fine without it. Believe me; I've never regretted not having the surgery.

Soon after we were out of the Army, another baby came along. I often thought I would have pursued a career earlier in my life had I been a little healthier, but that's just speculation. I was into motherhood too, and I ended up having five children! I had thought

about being a teacher instead of a librarian, but who knows? And
things have worked out very well for me. I've been working at the
library here at St. Cloud State University for five years. Before that,
I was at St. John's University for five years in their library. Then I
went to the public library for about four years. I took time out and
worked as a paralegal for another four years, which was a sad
mistake. Then I returned to the library. I was lucky to get back in.

I believe that I've had a successful career and a pretty normal life,
so I guess polio really hasn't affected my life experiences all that
much. Most people are not even aware that I've had it. I think that
what makes me think about it now is all of the publicity and writing
about the post-polio syndrome. I guess I'm alert for symptoms of
that. I have certainly felt none, except for fatigue, and I've wondered
if that is a part of it. I get tired a lot, and I think I fatigue more
easily than other people. I don't know; it's probably related to aging
too, but I think the polio has something to do with it as well.

My limp becomes more noticeable when I'm tired. My limp is not
painful or anything. It's just very noticeable. I don't have a smooth
walk. And I don't run at all. Maybe it's psychological, but I just
don't run. However, I do swim almost every day. I think that's
been very helpful. I've been swimming since 1977. I feel it energizes
me. The days I don't swim, I feel exhausted at night. If I do swim,
I feel okay. It's a strange thing.

My balance is bad, and I fall a lot. I tend to laugh it off, because
I've never hurt myself, yet I suppose one of these days I could really
get injured. One advantage of having poor balance is that it has
helped me to get a good parking space at work! I've told people I
don't have a good sense of balance, and I can't walk on slippery
sidewalks, so I have to park close to the library. They offered me a
handicapped spot, but I said it would be silly to hold down a
handicapped parking spot for eight hours a day. There must be
somebody else who needs it more than I do, and I think I'd feel
guilty if I parked there. I just need to get close enough to get in
without falling.

All in all though, I know that I was a very lucky polio victim. It
hasn't been a major part of my life. A lot of people don't even know
I've had polio, not that I've ever tried to hide it. It's just that my
disabilities are not very obvious, and they really don't keep me from
doing the things that I need to do.

I could have been a lot worse off. I have a friend who had polio.
He doesn't consider himself badly handicapped, but he is. When I

see that, I think if I had been younger and had more paralysis in my limbs it would have been much harder for me. So I consider myself extremely lucky.

Chapter 8

Old Timers

I doubt if the three individuals whose stories are included in this chapter would approve of the title. However, they are members of an ever declining group: those who had polio in the 1920's and 30's. Their stories give us a glimpse of what it was like to have had polio during those decades. It is interesting to note that none of the three recalls being hospitalized during his acute illness. In fact, they remember only home remedies and treatments. Yet, they recovered relatively well and went on to have successful lives. It is also interesting to note that in spite of having had polio more than 60 years ago, all three of these men continue to function relatively well.

Jack Dominik

I had polio in 1925. It affected my arms and legs, as well as my right hand. My left foot is a "drop foot." I can press down with it, but I can't lift it up. I can press down with my right foot a little and pick it up more easily. I have weakness in my right hand, and I can't lift either of my arms up over my head, not without holding them up. Other than that, I don't have any limitations. There were people who had it a lot worse than I did. They couldn't walk. I could always walk, and I could even run a little. But, at my age, I have more problems now, problems with balance and things like that.

Since I had polio when I was only three years old, I really don't remember much about the actual illness. My parents told me that I came down with it when we were coming back from the lake cottage where we spent our summers. Back then they didn't even call it polio; it was referred to as infantile paralysis.

I don't think that I went to the hospital, though I might have. To tell you the truth, I really only have one memory from the time that I was sick. I remember lying in my parents' bedroom, which was the only bedroom on the ground floor of the house, while my mother was out in the dining room. I recall that if I had my head turned one way and I wanted to turn it some other way, I would yell for my mom, and she would have to come in and turn my head for me. So I must have been pretty much completely paralyzed.

I also remember all of the strange medicines they bought for me to take. I recall my mom giving me rubdowns with goose grease. When I was given a bath, they were supposed to put salt in the water and make waves. I don't know what any of that was supposed to do. It sounds pretty hokey to me now. I also remember a medicine that came in a square can. It was kind of a yellowish color, and my mom would rub it on my legs. I think it was called Viavi. I'm not sure of how it would be spelled.

There were also some capsules that I took with meals, and I got a shot glass full of some liquid that I had to take with lunch every day. That was particularly vile tasting stuff. It was terrible! I remember hearing later that they had paid $300 for it. And that was 1928 or 1929, so that was really a lot of money back then. I'm not sure, but I think the stuff that I drank was bought from a door-to-door salesman. I suppose there were all sorts of medicines being sold back then that didn't really do a darn thing.

I remember my mom taking me to see doctors, but at that time I don't think anybody really knew what to do for you. Believe it or not, I think the salt water stuff was actually prescribed by a doctor. Maybe the goose grease was too. I'm not sure.

When I was in about third grade, I went down to a hospital in the Twin Cities and had an operation on my left leg. They separated the muscle that pulled up the right side of my foot and put part of it on the left side. It helped some. Instead of walking all the way over on the left side of my foot, I shifted over toward the right a little. I never could walk on the ball of my foot. I can still remember the doctors' names, Williamson and Cole. Williamson was an Englishman. I think he went back to England during World War II.

The next year, I went back and had surgery on the right leg. When they had operated on my left leg, they made three incisions, but on my right leg, they just did one long J-shaped incision down the outside of the leg and across the foot. They also talked about cutting the Achilles tendon so that I would be able to raise my left foot. I remember thinking about how much that would hurt. But fortunately, they never did it.

I remember that when I had the surgeries, or at least the first one, my mom stayed down there with me. Being the spoiled little brat that I was, I wouldn't stay down there by myself, so my mom was there for the three or four weeks that I was in the hospital recuperating. She slept on a cot in my room with me, but they couldn't give her any meals there. She only ate whatever I didn't eat from my meals, which wasn't very much. She should have just slapped me in the face and gone home!

I must have fussed and fumed until she agreed to stay. So my older sisters had to take care of everything back home. I'm not sure if she stayed both times or only for the first surgery. I really don't remember. I do remember, though, that the worst part of the surgeries was the itching and not being able to scratch because of the cast that they put on my leg. I got pretty good with using a knitting needle and sliding it down inside the cast and scratching where my hand couldn't reach.

I think that those operations were the last things that were done for me, at least medically. My dad bought a punching bag, and we put it down in the basement. Whenever I'd go down there, I'd play with that thing and punch and kick it around. But I never had any physical therapy or anything.

I never had to wear braces on my legs, but up until high school I always had to wear high-top shoes. They thought I needed the ankle support. That was before you could wear long pants, and those were the high shoes with the laces. I hated those things. By the time I got to high school, I guess they realized that wearing regular shoes would be more likely to help strengthen my ankles, so I finally got to wear Oxford shoes.

Other than my surgeries, I really don't think polio affected my childhood too much. I recall that when I was in grade school, this other boy and I sometimes didn't go out to recess with the other kids. He and I would stay in the classroom. Some nun was supposed to take care of us. Other than that, I don't remember anything special being done for me in grade school. I really didn't need any special help.

I did have some trouble writing, particularly with my right hand.

I think I wanted to write with my left hand. Maybe I was naturally left-handed, or maybe it was because of my disability. I don't know. But the nuns made me write with my right hand, which I do now. It would have been a lot easier if they had let me use my left hand; that's for sure.

I couldn't join in the running games and stuff like that. But I don't remember being teased or anything. In fact, some of the older kids used to look out for me. One boy used to walk home with me every day and make sure I got safely across a busy street. I don't think the nuns put him up to it or anything. I believe he just did it because he was a nice boy. I really didn't need his help because I was able to cross the street by myself, but he walked me home anyway.

Like I said, I really couldn't run very well, but I could swim a little. I remember one time out at Grand Lake when I was about six or seven years old. I was wading in the water up to my chest. The neighbors had this dog, and I was splashing water at the dog, and it would bite at the water. Well, the dog knocked me down, and there I was, lying on the bottom in about three feet of water looking up at the sun, and I couldn't get up. That's the last thing I remember. My sister ran out into the water and carried me back into the cottage. After that incident, I remember thinking that I'd better be more careful in the water.

My dad must have thought so too. Because when he bought some property on the Mississippi River and put in a swimming beach, he made a pen out in the water. That pen was for me. If I wanted to go swimming, I was supposed to stay in the pen.

I guess I really didn't learn my lesson, though. I remember the kids next door put up a rope on this big tree, and they would swing out over this bay and drop into the water and swim back. Well, I couldn't swim all that well, so I would just swing out on it and then swing back to shore. One time when I was swinging back, the rope broke. Fortunately, I landed in the soft mud right in between two rocks. Any further up and I would have been on the hard river bank, and any further down and I would have been in the deep water. Three chances out of four, I could have been hurt or killed, and I got the fourth. I thought that I must have had somebody special looking out for me. Anyway, after that incident, I truly did stop doing foolish stuff.

As far as my adult life, I really don't think polio had too much of an impact. Of course, polio did keep me out of the service during World War II. I remember going to the draft board with a couple of guys that I knew from high school, and the doctor told us to drop our pants. He just looked at me and wrote "obvious" on the form, and that was that.

I knew that I wasn't going to go, and I accepted it. There wasn't anything I could do about it. The only thing I felt badly about was that I couldn't be in the Air Corps. I've always liked flying. I had a cousin who was a flying instructor, so it would have been nice to have been in that. But I could have died in the war too, so I didn't feel that disturbed by it.

The only other impact is that I've always taken jobs that I could handle. When I was still in college out at Saint John's, I started a photographic finishing business with another guy, but before I graduated in 1945, the Army started using Saint John's for basic training of Air Corps recruits. Because of that and the war, there weren't too many civilian students out there, and they weren't teaching the courses I needed for an English degree. So I took a year off and looked around for a job that I could handle. I ended up taking a job at a radio station, but some guy came back out of service, and I was replaced. After that, I went back and finished my senior year of college.

After college, I got a job teaching English, but I only did that for one year because the monks started coming back after the war, and they didn't need me. Then I went to work for the Sentinel, which at that time was publishing the weekly newspaper in St. Cloud. I was originally hired just to be a photographer, but then they found out I had been an English major in college. So they made me be a reporter too. Well, the salary that I was getting paid was all right for just being a photographer, but when they made me a reporter too, they didn't give me a raise. After about a year there, I just decided that I wasn't going to do both of those jobs for that salary, and I took a job as a copywriter for an advertising company. I ended up staying there for 12 years.

I had to change jobs again though, because the owner was going to sell the agency, and I wasn't sure what that would mean for me. So I took a job in advertising at the Saint John's Liturgical Press, and I worked there until just recently when I retired.

I was always just a copywriter there. If it hadn't been for polio, I probably would have done a lot more, like going to conventions and setting up booths, going overseas with people, and so on. But not being able to help with stuff like that, I just remained a copywriter. I think that was the only effect polio had on my career there.

I've been very fortunate in that I haven't had any of the post-polio problems that I've heard about. I think it's been over 60 years since I've seen a doctor about anything to do with my polio. I have had other medical problems, of course, but I don't believe they're related to my polio. I had pneumonia, kidney stones, and a heart attack. Then about two years ago I had a pacemaker put in because I kept having dizzy spells and would pass out and fall down. The pacemaker took care of that.

I have had more problems walking as I've gotten older. Whether it's due to my drop foot dropping more or not, I don't know. I've fallen more in the last five or six years than in the last 40 or 50 put together, so I've got to be a little more careful.

I did see a physical therapist when I was having the dizzy spells, and she tried to have me move my legs this way and that way, but I couldn't do most of the things she wanted. Later, I got a call from some guy in town who makes braces, and he asked if there was any way he could help. Well, the only thing I could think of would be some kind of plastic thing that would fit on the back of my leg and go under my left foot so that as soon as I lifted the leg it would raise my toe. However, if it was too strong, it might throw my knee out. Then I'd fall every step. So, I just said, "The heck with it. I'll just get along the way I've been doing all this time." If nothing else, I'm used to it!

Charles A. Stone

I was born in 1924 in the northern Minnesota town of Park Rapids. My dad was the Forest Ranger Supervisor for that area, and my parents also were in the hotel and resort business there. About 1930, probably sometime during the summer, I contracted polio. I guess no one was sure what I had until after I got over the acute stage of the illness. It was only after I was well enough to get out of bed, and I was dragging my left leg, that it was determined I'd had polio.

As far as I know, I was never hospitalized during my bout with polio. Rather, I was treated at home. My mom was a registered nurse, and though I don't believe she had ever heard of Sister Kenny and her treatment approach, mom had always been an advocate of wet hot packs and massage. So when I was in bed having pain and discomfort, she literally spent weeks hot packing and massaging those areas of my body that hurt. Later, I learned that Sister Kenny had developed a treatment method resembling what my mom had done with me.

I ended up recovering quite well in that I was left only with tightness and, perhaps, a little weakness in my left leg. That leg was always a little smaller, and as I grew, my left foot was maybe a size smaller than my right. I don't know if this is true or not, but I've always attributed my excellent recovery to my mother and her use of hot packs and massage.

My parents didn't want me to be held back by my polio, so for several years they concealed the fact that I'd had it. It wasn't until I was going out for sports as I started high school that my father and mother finally told me. They were concerned that I might get hurt because my older brother had gotten injured playing football. So my parents decided to sit down and talk to me, and it was then that I learned what I'd had.

After learning this, I began to understand why certain things had always been a little different for me. For instance, I understood why I had so many cramps in my left leg and why the little girl who lived next door was able to skate faster than I could. I also understood why my left leg would tend to unexpectedly fly off my bike pedal when I'd be riding down the road.

So I didn't go out for athletics in high school. Instead, I found other ways to express myself. I designed and built the prize winning homecoming float two years in a row. And since I had always had an interest in airplanes and aviation, I spent a lot of time building model airplanes and reading about flying. I think I must have read every book about airplanes that was available at that time.

My interest in aviation led me to enlist in the Army Air Corps during World War II. In April of 1943, just prior to my high school graduation, I went down to the Federal Building in the Twin Cities and went through the exam process to try and get into the Aviation Cadet Program. As I started through the process, I was interviewed by a flight surgeon, and I revealed to him that I'd had polio. Now, at that time, the difference in diameter between my left and right legs wasn't very noticeable. There was only a slight difference, so I was able to snow the doctors with how physically fit I was. Yet, when I told him about my history of polio, he immediately said, "Well, I don't think we can take you." So I turned on the heat and begged him to let me try, and he finally gave in and did let me try. I suppose he was thinking that they'd find some other reason to wash me out.

After I finished all the tests, he sat down with me again and pulled out the monthly manual that they were issuing to flight surgeons giving the exams. He said, "Here son, I'll explain why we can't take you." He started paging through the manual looking for the section that excluded anyone with a history of polio from being a pilot, and he couldn't find it. He paged through the thing three or four times, and he was just getting frantic. Finally, the guy said, "I'll be damned! They must have forgotten to put that in this month." I told him about my life-long interest in aviation and being a pilot. By this time he was getting exasperated. He looked at me and said, "You're never going to make it, but I'm going to let you try." So I got my chance, which was all I was asking for.

After finishing high school that spring, I went right into the Army Air Corps as an Aviation Cadet. However, by that time, the pilot training programs were getting pretty full, so because of a number of delays, and going from one facility to another, it took me 19 months to finally graduate. A lot of guys washed out, but I was able to hang in there and become a pilot. I've often wished that the flight surgeon who told me I'd never make it had been there to see me graduate!

My graduation day turned out to be bittersweet, however. On that very day, it was announced that our entire class was to be sent for further training to be flight engineers on B-29's. They had been losing too many B-29's in combat, and they thought that by adding a third pilot as a flight engineer, they might improve the combat performance of that aircraft. It had been my dream to be a fighter pilot, and that's what I had been training for, but I had no choice but to follow orders and become a flight engineer. I completed that training and graduated with a second air crew rating.

From there, I was sent to Texas for combat crew training. However, I never actually got into combat. While I was there, they dropped the atomic bomb, and everything at that base just came to a screeching halt. Nothing flew; nobody fixed anything; and my dream of having a career as an Air Force pilot was just going down the tubes. I ended up being sent from one holding area to another with nothing to do. Finally, after months of being in limbo, I was at Grand Island, Nebraska, and they called us all together. We were told that our outfit was going to Alaska to fly long range weather missions over the North Pole. I had the choice to do that or to get out. After thinking it over, I decided to get out.

I returned to Park Rapids and took over the operation of my parents' hotel/resort. It was there that I met my wife, Nell. We got married in October, 1946, and the two of us ran the hotel until 1951 when I took a voluntary recall into the Air Force. The resort business was becoming increasingly difficult, and I felt that I had never really gotten a chance to fulfill my ambitions to fly during World War II. After talking it over with my wife, I called an Air Force officer who had spent some time fishing at our resort. They needed pilots again because of the Korean War, and he put my name in for recall. I got orders which would have assigned me to be a radar officer, but I called headquarters and told them I wanted to fly. That was why I had gotten back in, so they changed my orders and sent me to flight instructors school for a six-week course.

After completing that, I went to Texas where I was a B-25 advanced flight instructor. I had never flown a twin-engine plane before, let alone a B-25, but after only three flights to check me out, I began teaching advanced flight students and learning the aircraft myself at the same time. I volunteered for combat duty, but didn't get it. The Air Force felt I was more valuable as a flight instructor.

After about two years there, I was transferred to another base in Texas for photo/recon training. I then became a B-29 Aircraft Commander and was sent to Japan where we flew classified missions doing electronic and some photographic reconnaissance. It was rather primitive equipment compared to now, but it was exciting. We'd get Russian fighters on our wings every once in a while.

I did my one-year tour there, and then was transferred back to the United States. It was about this time, maybe even a little earlier, that I started to have these weird occurrences in my life that were inexplicable then, but as I learned much later, were probably polio-related. I'm not saying everything that happened was due to polio, but some of it certainly was.

I was starting to have physical difficulties while I was stationed in Japan, but I was able to cope with them. However, in the summer of 1954, I was sent to flight school at McConnell Air Force Base to learn to fly the B-47. While I was completing that training, I was exercising one night to try to keep myself in shape, and I developed severe back spasms that just literally tied me in knots. I'd never experienced that before, and in retrospect, I can see now that they were probably due to the tightness and weakness in my left leg and may have been early post-polio symptoms. The spasms persisted for a few weeks until they finally backed off enough to allow me to make it through my combat crew training and become a B-47 Aircraft Commander.

I was stationed in Lincoln, Nebraska and commanded a numbered

SAC bomber that had assigned targets in the Soviet Union. Two days before we were to fly to England for a temporary mission, which was to require a night take off and aerial refueling, my back spasms reoccurred. I just went to my knees and had knots in my back. The next morning I could hardly manage to put on my flight suit. My back problems really presented me with a dilemma. Should I admit to my problems and possibly get scrubbed from the mission, or should I try to hide my condition and just go on like nothing had happened? I swallowed my pride and decided that I needed to go to the hospital and at least get the situation checked out. The flight surgeon I saw there seemed to think I was goofing off or perhaps my problems were due to the stress of the mission, so he just told me to take some APC pills.

The spasms eased off enough that I managed to get my plane and crew ready for the mission, and we took off for England. As we were descending to rendezvous with the refueling tanker, the spasms came back to the extent that I had great difficulty using my left foot to control the rudder. We had a terrible time refueling; the boom kept popping out because my plane's refueling system was defective, and we kept ejecting the boom. As it turned out, we couldn't get enough fuel to make it to our alternate base where we would have had to land if the weather was bad in England. To be safe, we had to turn around and fly back to Nebraska. Within 24 hours, however, the refueling system was fixed. We took off again, and along with two other planes that had experienced problems on the initial flight, we headed back for England. This time everything went according to plan, and we made it.

We stayed on alert in England for several months, making practice runs down to Africa. My back pain persisted, and by now, the problems were serious enough that they were threatening my status as an aircraft commander. I talked to the flight surgeon again, but he just interpreted what I had told him to mean that I wanted to get a medical discharge from the Air Force, which wasn't true at all.

I made it through my time in England and flew back to Nebraska. My squadron commander flew back with me in case I had any problems. We made it back okay, but my back problems continued, particularly when I had to be on my feet for any length of time. I was in and out of contact with doctors, and the Air Force was starting to wonder what to do with me. Eventually I was taken off combat crew duty and given the assignment of heading a program to solve some survival equipment problems we were experiencing with the B-47.

Soon thereafter, I became the Wing Ground Training Officer, and later the Base Training Officer.

About that same time, the Air Force came up with a program that would allow reserve officers like me to convert to regular Air Force status. I really wanted to do that, but before they would let me, I was sent to be evaluated by a civilian neurologist. He gave me a clean bill of health and said I was fit for flight duty. Therefore, I was allowed to convert my status. However, my back problems recurred periodically, and in 1959 I was sent to the V.A. Hospital. They put me in a body cast for a while, but that didn't help, so finally, they decided to do exploratory surgery. They intended to fuse my spine, but ended up only carving off some calcium deposits that were pinching off my nerves. I don't know if those calcium deposits were polio-related, but I do know that my body tends to use calcium differently.

After I recovered from the surgery, I was transferred to 2nd Air Force Headquarters at Barksdale AFB, Louisiana to manage a variety of training programs. During this assignment, I was again able to pass my flight physical and returned to flight status. While there, I developed a plan of action to solve existing shooting training problems. This plan was eventually published as a manual and caught the interest of the Director of Training at the Pentagon in Washington D.C. Soon thereafter, I was transferred to the Pentagon where I served as manager of the Air Force General Military Training Program.

Though I was under a lot of stress and working very hard, I managed to do the jobs I'd been assigned quite well. However, the stress and long hours finally caught up with me, and in 1964 I became extremely ill. I got up to go to work on a Monday morning, and I had a partial loss of vision and problems with balance. I got a ride to work and checked into the Air Force Dispensary at the Pentagon, and that started a never ending series of physical evaluations. By this time, my left leg was noticeably smaller, and combining that and my current symptoms with my history of back pain, they didn't know what to think.

I was evaluated at Andrews Air Force Base, and then I spent about six weeks at Walter Reed Hospital in Washington D.C. where I was given all sorts of tests. I ended up getting tentative diagnoses that were basically just shots in the dark. They told me they thought I had everything from an inner ear problem to encephalitis to a brain tumor. Finally, in January of 1965, a doctor told me that though they didn't know for sure, they thought I probably had ALS (amyotrophic lateral sclerosis), and I'd be dead in about two years! I thought if that was the case, I sure didn't want to spend those two years sitting around in a hospital. I decided that I wanted to go back to work.

At that time, I only needed about four more years until I'd be able to retire with 20 years of service. So I called a general with whom I had worked, and he intervened on my behalf and managed to get me out of the medical retirement system. I put in two more years at the Pentagon, and throughout those two years, I continued to have weird symptoms. My balance was still bad, and my leg kept getting skinnier. I also started to get fasciculations (jerking motions), particularly in the calf of my left leg. Of course, I continued to get medical evaluations, including brain wave analyses, to check the progression of my condition. Time was moving on, but I was hanging in there, doing my job. Finally, a neurologist I was seeing told me he didn't think I had ALS after all, which was a relief. However, he also told me that he didn't know what I had, and all they could do was keep watching me.

In the spring of 1966, I was transferred to Naples, Italy where I served as the Executive Officer for an Italian General assigned to NATO. I had some very bad allergic reactions there, which I later learned may have been made worse by my history of polio, but I did my job and completed my two years there.

I retired from the Air Force as a lieutenant colonel in 1968 and moved to Flagstaff, Arizona where I enrolled at Northern Arizona University. I chose to go far away from Minnesota because I thought that if my body was going to fall apart, I sure didn't want it to happen in my home state. But my body didn't fall apart, and I ended up graduating from college with my daughter in 1973. We then moved to Little Falls, Minnesota where I started a woodworking, photographic, and display business. In 1978 I accepted a position as Manager of the Lindbergh Historical Site, where I worked until I retired in 1990.

During the time I was working at the Lindbergh Site, I attended two post-polio seminars, and they were a revelation to me. I found myself surrounded by people who'd also had strange things happen to their bodies. I learned that the deterioration of my left leg was due to post-polio syndrome. I also learned that my back spasms and even some of my other problems may also have been polio-related. Since attending those seminars, I've been careful to take better care of myself and not overdo.

My left leg continues to get a little thinner and tighter every year, and now it's less than half the diameter of my right leg. I have to stretch and exercise, but I'm able to do most of the things that I need and want to do. I still walk without the need of a brace or cane, and my wife and I keep busy running our family business, which provides educational consulting and fabrication services to non-profit organizations.

As I look back on my life, I can see now that my hard driving personality and workaholic attitudes were overcompensations for my disability. I've always felt that I needed to be a hard charger and not show any signs of weakness. I also know that these attitudes contributed to the success I've had throughout my life. So, as I reflect on my career and my experiences, I do so with few, if any, regrets.

Bill Van Cleve

I'm Bill, and I'm four months shy of my 68th birthday. My background is pretty simple. I am the eldest of five children, and I was born in a little suburb of Newark, New Jersey back in the spring of 1926. I had polio somewhere in my 9th or early 10th year, about 1935. I know that it was in the summertime because I learned later that I was thought to have contracted it at the large public swimming pool in nearby Olympic Park. My sisters and friends and I would swim in that pool for three hours every other day in June, July, and August because the park was so close. We had to pay a 10 cent fee to get in as I recall.

I don't remember when or how I was diagnosed. Obviously we had a family doctor. We had the same person for many years, and he must've taken whatever measures he could to make the diagnosis. He then told my parents that I had polio, and they told me. The little I can remember about the illness itself is that I felt extremely ill. I was nauseous, hot, achy, and feverish. I was not put in the hospital. It was thought only necessary that I stay in bed. I'm not sure how long I was in bed, but it was long enough so that I had to drop out of the fifth grade.

I was in a parochial school that was a part of our parish, and I think most of that year I had a home teacher provided by the public school system. My regular teacher, Sister Mary Leonie, wrote me every week or so to see how I was doing, and she told me what she was doing with the class. Maybe once a month or so, she had the class write me letters which would be put in this big envelope, and one of my sisters would bring it home to me.

The most vivid memory I have of the actual illness is when I was paralyzed in my legs and arms. I think that with the aid of someone I was able to "hobble" into the bathroom. I don't recall being so confined to bed that I literally had to use a bedpan, but I know I ate all my meals in bed, so maybe I did have to use a bedpan, at least for a while.

I don't remember if I got any medications or anything, but at some point after this initial attack subsided, my mother learned of the Sister Kenny method. Many people, of course, knew of my illness and gave my parents advice about what to do. So maybe somebody suggested that method to her. I don't know, but I have a distinct memory in which I can see myself lying in this double bed in an oblong kind of room with one window behind the bed and my mother coming in and smiling and lifting up first one, then the other leg, and bending it slightly and doing the same with my arms. My mom never put the hot compresses on me like they did in the 1940's and 50's. She just would bend and lift my limbs. I didn't even know the name Sister Kenny at the time. My mother just did these things, and later, considerably later, when I was older and we would revisit the early days and so forth, it was then that I learned it was the Sister Kenny method she was following.

Bending those limbs was very painful. I cried, and of course, it was hard for her to see a 10-year-old child crying. She would also give me a pretty sturdy rub with alcohol all over the back region and thighs, hips, and so forth. I have very little memory of pain and misery though. Instead, I have memories of spending my time building model airplanes with the old sticks and the slides in the wings with the slats and then covering them with tissue paper. After that, I would wet the paper slightly, and as it dried it would stretch real tight on the wings. Of course, they had elastic bands and a propeller. I built a lot of those. I also read formidably. By that I mean that my family always rewarded scholastic accomplishment. All report cards were scrutinized, and grades were commented on, so reading just seemed like the natural thing for me to do.

I guess I was in bed for about a year, but I don't know precisely. Both my father and mother are dead now, so I couldn't ask them. My sister Virginia supposedly had a slight touch of polio too, but apparently it was mostly just fever and aches. No actual paralysis occurred. But as far as my recovery, I believe that in something under a year I had recovered enough that I was able to navigate unaided and without crutches or anything. The only residue of my illness was flat feet with the tendency for my toes to point slightly outward when I walked.

Because of the problems with my feet, I was taken to Orange Orthopedic Hospital in East Orange, New Jersey, and the doctors there said, "Gee, we can fix this up. With a slice in the inner side of the arch we can remove a little bit of the tendon there, and that will cause the arch to curve up again." So at some point, say maybe a couple of years after this initial polio episode, I was admitted to Orange Orthopedic for these two very simple, very routine operations, which were done simultaneously. But unfortunately, the surgeries didn't go as well as they had predicted, and my right foot developed an osteomyelitis bone infection. It began to drain both from a sore where the original surgery was and from the upper part of the ankle. It had to have a bandage removed daily and thrown away. My foot had to be washed, have some salve put on it, and then be re-wrapped. It stank terribly.

For a while, it didn't impede putting on a normal shoe, but this problem persisted for some four or five years with the result that my right ankle became somewhat weakened. It became short in length by about an inch and a half, and now there's about a two inch difference from my "normal" foot.

If that operation had taken place today, and I got an infection in a hospital like I did back then, I'm sure we would be expected to sue the hospital. But people didn't do that back then, and really, I have very little sympathy for all the various law suits that occur today.

Anyway, I spent several months in the hospital because of that bone infection, and I can remember being in a large ward with perhaps 10 beds and one nurse. There probably was a night and a day nurse, and I remember "Ma Hunley" as one of the nurses. I can still see her face very clearly. She reminded me of an aunt or grandma perhaps: firm, but kind and caring. I can also remember that my fellow patients, all male, ranged from a man who I thought was 60, but he might've only been 40, to a boy named Walter, whose entire body was encased in plaster. He had a big bar between his two legs which were spread apart, and his crotch was open. It seemed to me that his legs were spread eagle. If I remember right, the cast even covered his head. So Walter was plaster from head to foot. I was less aware of the others, but I think there were 9 or 10 beds. We would have a 35mm movie on Sundays, and I really looked forward to that. There was nothing like television. There may have been a radio that they brought in so we could hear the "Lone Ranger" or something.

After I got out of the hospital, I must've been doing excess walking because I remember twice falling and breaking my right knee and having to go on crutches because I had a heavy plaster cast from my ankle up to my hip. That wasn't fun. And to make matters worse, I had to miss school and have home teaching again. I remember being in a wheelchair, and I remember being wheeled out onto our front open porch which faced south, so it had nice sun. I remember a little Sears radio, which cost about $10, and that was a lot of money back in the 1930's in depression-ridden America, on which I listened to the "Romance of Helen Trent" and all the other soaps while I would sit out on that porch.

Anyway, I didn't start wearing a built-up shoe until late in high school when it seemed the easiest way to deal with the limp that I had developed. The first couple of pairs were made up by an orthopedic shoe place, and they were ugly looking, and I felt terrible about wearing them. They really called attention to themselves. I just hated those sons of ..., and I haven't worn them since somewhere in college. During college, I had lifts made of leather, rubber, or whatever was durable enough and light enough. I'm not self-conscious about how I look, and haven't been for 30 years, but when I was young I was more sensitive about my appearance. I wanted to look nice, and in my case, handsome and nice. You naturally feel that way during adolescence.

I was, of course, disqualified from military service in World War II. When I was 18 and in high school, I remember going down to the gym with the other boys in my junior class and stripping to our shorts. The U.S. Navy recruiting team was there, and we went through this physical, and somehow I made myself believe that our country needed me enough that they would ignore this slightly smaller leg. I could run fairly well although I'd never played any sports. I chose to think that was a choice. I would much rather do photography, debating, journalism, or whatever. But, needless to say, the Navy said, "We're not taking you with that short foot," and I was just crushed. I almost felt like I had been drummed out of the male corps or something. I might say that I think because of the war, the scout troop that I had been in since I was in grade school made me scout master. It was probably because all the older guys were out fighting the bad guys. But anyway, one effect of polio was initially the great disappointment that I couldn't become a soldier, sailor, or whatever in World War II. Later on though, I thanked God because, while I might've won a medal and so forth, I also might've ended up dead or severely injured in that war.

So I wasn't going to be in the service, and when I started high school, I never intended to go to college. I followed the college-prep curriculum, but I expected to get a blue-collar job, although we didn't really think of work as blue-collar/white-collar back then. I was going to work in a tool room where I could become a tool-and-die maker. I had part-time jobs throughout high school, and that income helped pay for the things I wanted that my parents couldn't afford to buy me. I also paid board during the last two years of high school from my earnings as a truck driver and a soda clerk and later as a tool room assistant in a large defense factory. But then my mother heard that the state of New Jersey had a rehabilitation program, primarily for people who either through disease, birth defect, or accident had severe physical handicaps, that would teach them a trade so they could be self-supporting. Somehow this woman, who herself was only a high school graduate, desired that I would go on to college.

My father died of cancer when I was a senior in high school, and I thought, "Well, now more than ever, I will go to work and help my mother support my four younger sisters and brother." I finished high school in three and a half years thinking that the quicker I could graduate, the quicker I could get to work. But my mom learned that the state rehabilitation commission might pay for something like teacher training. There was a college that was a nickel-streetcar ride away. This college, the Newark State Teacher's College, would've been all right, but she somehow managed to get me admitted to Rutgers, which was 40 miles away, and where I had to stay and have all the wonderful pleasures of living in a dormitory. I entered in the Fall of 1945 with a face full of acne and a very limited knowledge of the real world because of my parochial school background. There were guys at Rutgers who had heard shots fired. They talked about their war exploits quite a bit, and I was stunned at the kind of world that was opening up before my eyes.

While I was in college, people would notice that I limped, and they'd often ask, "Did you hurt yourself? You seem to limp a little," and I always do limp a little. Early on I probably told the polio story more because it was my "war wound." I didn't have the war wound that I wished I did have. Now I'm glad I don't have one, but when you're 18 or 19 and surrounded by warriors, you wish you were a warrior too. But anyway, I ended up getting an excellent college education because of the fact that I had polio.

The state support for me was more generous than the support given to a hungry, World War II G.I., and believe me, that was generous. A single G.I. received 95 bucks a month, tuition, books, and support at any college in the country that would take them. So, if they got into expensive Harvard University, the government would even pay for that. If they got into a state, six-dollars-a-credit college, they'd pay that plus the 95 bucks, and it went up to $125 if you were married, plus so much more for each kid. But I got more out of the state of New Jersey than a single, World War II veteran, and I'm very grateful to the New Jersey State Rehabilitation Program that was legislated somewhere in the 1930's, and to Mrs. Leah B. Mack who was my social worker. I had to write to her every semester and visit her annually and send her my transcript. She took a real interest in my progress down there, from courses and grades to my student activities and even my dating life. It was marvelous. I was in the School of Education, which in those days took a very small bite out of your four years. Less than 20% of all the credits were required for education courses. So I was able to get a full English and history major plus an education minor as you would call it today.

I'm elaborating on this so much because it changed my life. No one in our large extended family had attended college except my father during the 1930's, when he went to night classes at the Newark College of Engineering. I'd say to myself, "Well, why am I doing this? I'm supposed to go out and work; it's the right thing for the oldest to do," and my mother would say, "Your father would have wanted it, and I want it." So you might say that one impact polio had on my life is that it resulted in me having the opportunity to get a college education.

Now, another main effect of my having had polio is that a lot of attention was paid to me. There were no social services that were available to help us through this, at least not when I had the initial illness or when I had surgery. So my mom had to do a lot of things for me, and I think I got used to being the center of attention. I got used to people doing things for me. "Could I get something for you? What do you want?" I became very self-centered. My sisters, whom I love and now love me, said I was unbearable. I would get funny books or comic books to read and put them under my covers. My sisters would come in, "Got any funny books?" I'd tell them that I didn't. I was just being mean. I had a radio that my Aunt Madeline gave me, and my sisters would come and say, "Can I listen with you?" And I wouldn't let them listen, so I got spoiled and self-centered and also got a fairly strong sense that people should do whatever I asked them to do. I became a controlling and insensitive kind of person.

I'm an alcoholic, and I have been an alcoholic since somewhere in my late teens when I went to college. I don't know how much of the personality distortion occurred because of my having polio and being bed-ridden and treated special. However, I can't help but wonder if that laid the foundation for over-reliance on drinking and the tendency to medicate the frustrations or the disappointments or to help celebrate the triumphs. But by the time I was married in my mid-20's, I was unable to go through a day without at least a drink. By the time I was 30, I needed a couple of drinks, and so it went. However, it wasn't until I was in my early 50's, around 1979, that I went into treatment for my alcoholism.

Believe me, entering treatment was certainly not voluntary. My wife arranged an intervention, and she didn't tell me about it in a friendly tone. I quickly agreed to the intervention because I was tired of her nagging and chipping away. I felt that she'd never enjoyed a drink because she didn't know what the good things in life were. When I say that, I'm speaking like the drunk I was. So when she said, "We want you to go in the hospital and have this drinking checked out," I thought, "Sure, because I know I'm not an alcoholic. How could I be the registrar of a university and have all these powerful friends if I was an alcoholic?"

Well, they finally got that fool notion out of my head, and I'm still today thankfully and gratefully sober and a member of AA. Now, what role in the etiology of my alcoholism polio played, God will someday tell me, should she choose to do so. I do know it certainly contributed to my being arrogant and spoiled. I hope the people I treated badly when I was that way have had the grace to forgive me.

Do I think my life would have been different if I didn't have polio? Well sure, but how different? I'd like to think that maybe I wouldn't have taken so long to grow up. I think I was immature well into my married life. I was immature in thinking that everybody should defer to me and that I was something special and that my voice and views counted more than anyone else's. I had pretty strong defects in areas like that. I think it would've been good, perhaps, if I had sort of a "hard-knocks" type of experience, even playing football or something and getting pushed around a little by bigger, stronger kids, but that never happened to me. In that sense I think it might've been different.

I think the brains I have are, of course, the heritage of my parents. And I think that even if I had not initially gone to college because of the need to work, I probably would have sooner or later found my way there because by the 1950's, and certainly today, there is a strong message that college is the way to get ahead in life.

Am I sad or glad that I had it? Well, sad in the sense that it gave me some bad habits to overcome, but life is learning to overcome your bad habits. It's learning to outgrow your infantile behaviors, and I certainly still have a ways to go, but I think I'm further along than I was, say 20 or 30 years ago. And I've got another 20 years, God willing, to get rid of the rest.

I'm told by a therapist with whom I work that I do tend to put myself down more than I should, and maybe that's related to having had polio. I was a bright, interesting, stimulating talker. I could remember and summarize what I'd read. I could pull a couple of interesting questions to yack about, so I think I deserved some of the praise and attention. But I've always thought that I got more than I should have because of my illness.

Are there other effects from having had polio? Well, I think I've always rooted for the underdog. In my later years, I've become somewhat politically conservative, but I'm still a sucker for somebody who's really been dealt bad cards by life. I was a New Dealer, when I first learned what the term meant, and Roosevelt was one of my heros. I didn't vote for Roosevelt, of course, because he died before I could vote, but I've been to his home in Warm Springs, and I've even been to his summer place up off the coast of Maine.

Another great hero I remember from those years was a man named Fred Smythe Jr. Smythe was the son of a very well-to-do family who was so paralyzed in his lungs that he had to be in an iron lung. I guess that was not uncommon for polio cases. His family enabled him, even with this piece of baggage, to go to places like China. He eventually married. I still have in my mind this picture of Smythe's hand holding the girl's hand from the iron lung as the preacher said the words.

So, I guess you could say that my having had polio influenced who my heros were. And I do think some of my social and political views and my "pull for the underdog attitude" have been greatly influenced by polio. However, it's interesting, and this may sound like a contradiction, though I don't see it as one. I find myself reacting negatively today to so-called disabled or physically challenged people.

I often use the term derisively. I have made cracks about "crippled" people parking spaces. When I see the expensive adjustments to physical terrain that have been made by places like the colleges where I worked in order to benefit perhaps one person in a year or one person in a week or whatever, I get angry. Maybe it's because nothing like that was done for any of us when we had polio. After all, I had to manage without any of those things when I was in a wheelchair, so perhaps, it's just jealousy. But, for whatever reason, the notion that all of society should stand aside for those who are handicapped or disabled or challenged, is one to which I am not too sympathetic. Nor do I approve of the huge expenditures for the disabled that are made out of the public treasury. And like I said, I don't know if that's because I had polio or not.

Trying to put all of this in perspective, if you were to say, "Bill, I'm going to let you be born again. We'll move back the clock to the 1920's, and you can change one aspect of your life, any one aspect." I know that I'd want the same parents. I'd want to live in the same economic and religious status that I lived in. I am married to the same person I first proposed to, and I am extremely happily married. I have four children, of whom I am extremely proud, so I certainly wouldn't change any of that. But I would hope that I would not have become so god-damned fond of alcohol. That's the one thing I would change, because I not only hurt myself, but I hurt a lot of other people over the more than 30 years that I was a drunk.

As far as the polio, I see that as one of the various "bad" things that have happened in my life. However, it's much less a bad thing than the alcohol.

Chapter 9

Complete (or Almost Complete) Recovery

Although most of those we interviewed for this project were left with some residual disability as a result of contracting polio, several seem to have recovered completely or, at least, nearly so. The stories of five of these individuals are included in this chapter. Because they recovered so completely, these interviewees were spared the ordeals of braces, surgeries, and additional hospitalizations. Therefore, compared to most of the other stories that appear in this book, these are relatively brief.

In some cases this recovery occurred in spite of significant initial paralysis and dire prognoses. Yet, there seems to be nothing extraordinary in so far as the initial or follow-up treatment these individuals received. The reason that they recovered so well is simply another one of polio's mysteries.

It is also interesting to note that, in spite of their excellent recoveries, even these individuals are not immune to concerns about post-polio syndrome. While all five whose stories appear in this chapter continue to do relatively well, two report having aches, pains, and other symptoms that they worry may be signs of post-polio syndrome.

Millie Teders

In the fall of 1942, I was nine years old and had just begun the fourth grade. We lived on a farm, and I had helped my dad in a sorghum field over the weekend. I had gotten wet, chilled, and overtired. When I went to school on Monday, I developed a severe headache during the afternoon. We always walked to and from school (almost three miles each way), and I had to walk home that day even though I was not feeling well.

The next morning my headache was gone, and I was sure I was feeling well enough to go to school, so I walked there with my brother. By 10:00 that morning, however, I had a splitting headache again. The teacher gave me an aspirin, but it didn't help much. I was forced to stay in school all day because the school didn't have a telephone, and neither did my parents. At the end of the school day, I literally dragged myself home, and by the time I got there, I was vomiting and felt terribly ill.

I went to bed when I got home and slept until the next morning. When I woke up, I had a terribly stiff neck along with the other symptoms, so my folks drove me to the doctor. The doctor checked me over and found a spot on one lung, so he treated me with sulfa for pneumonia. He suspected polio, but he checked my reflexes, and they still worked.

I was put in the hospital in Staples, Minnesota, and every day the doctor would have me sit on the side of the bed so he could check my reflexes. Then he would have me walk. On the third day I was there, he came in to see me, and I no longer had reflexes when he tapped my knees with the hammer. When he got me up to walk, I collapsed. My legs would no longer hold me up.

My doctor was sure now that I had polio, and he felt the Sister Kenny treatment would be very helpful for me. This was a very new treatment at that time, and a lot of the doctors were not enlightened enough to use it. Instead, they were mostly putting affected limbs in casts. But, that only made the muscles wither, and the arm or leg became completely useless. The only hospitals that offered the Sister Kenny treatment at that time were Gillette Hospital and the University of Minnesota Hospital in Minneapolis. My doctor called down to the hospitals, but both were full and were not accepting patients. He recommended that my parents drive me to the University Hospital in the middle of the night, feeling that they would not turn a sick child away.

He was right, and they did accept me. The next day, they did a very painful spinal tap to find if I had polio or spinal meningitis. After that, I spent four painful months in a ward with seven other polio patients. I was treated with hot packs, and they stretched my muscles three times a day. I was paralyzed on my whole left side, even my face. The time in the hospital was very lonely for me, as my parents couldn't afford to come and see me very often.

I have many other memories of my time in the hospital. These range from bad food to wheelchair races. During one of our races, I tried to maneuver through a very narrow space and knocked a couple of tiles off the wall, so the nurses put a stop to the wheelchair races. Of course, the bad food never stopped. I remember that the jello was so rubbery, we used to play catch with it!

Incidentally, I met Sister Kenny a couple of times when I was in the hospital. She stretched my legs and showed the nurses how to do it correctly. That didn't endear her to me at the time because the stretching was quite painful.

I got out of the hospital at the end of January and had to use crutches for about six months. A few months after I got home, I started developing nervous mannerisms and twitching of the muscles. I ended up back in the University Hospital where I was diagnosed as having chorea or St. Vitus's dance. I guess it was not uncommon for that disease to follow polio. I was in bed for six months this time, as chorea affects the heart like rheumatic fever, and you need complete bed rest for a long time.

I couldn't live at home during this time, because I had five brothers and sisters, and I was supposed to have things very quiet. An aunt and uncle took me in to live with them for five months. All together, I was out of school for nearly two full years, but I was able to study at home and eventually caught up with my class.

Looking back on all this, I feel very fortunate because I've been able to live quite a normal life after all my early trauma. I'm married, and I have four children and eleven grandchildren. Thanks to a smart doctor and the Sister Kenny treatment, I recovered very well, and the aftereffects of polio have been slight compared to those of a lot of people I know. I have a slight limp; my left leg is a little bit smaller and has a tight heel cord, and I'm very stiff when I get up in the morning or after sitting for a while. But these problems I can live with.

I think my illness affected my family a good deal. My dad farmed a very small farm. He had a few dairy cattle, some pigs, and chickens. He was a very hardworking, proud man, and he had to beg for money from the county to take care of me and pay the hospital bills. He spent years paying the county back by cutting brush along roads and under telephone lines. He also worked on a railroad and, of course, continued farming. He would never accept charity without paying it back. It seems to me that's a far cry from the attitudes of many people today.

Elaine Lodermeier

I was 16 years old in the spring of 1945. I remember that at the end of the school year our teacher told us about polio. She warned us about going swimming and getting bad sunburns because it was thought that those things might make you more susceptible to polio. Of course, being 16 years old, I didn't listen. I went out and did all those things anyway. I went swimming and then took a boat out. I fell asleep in the boat and got a bad sunburn on my back. It was all blistered. That happened at the end of June. Then, the first week in July, I developed tonsillitis. It seemed like I got that every July.

Towards the middle of July, I started getting really sick. My mom put me to bed, and I remember that I kept coughing up phlegm. Then I started getting delirious, and I would see cracks in the ceiling and other things that weren't really there. Finally, my mom took me to the doctor, and he said I had an abscess in my throat. He suggested that I take a raw egg and try to swallow it. The egg went straight down, and then I couldn't swallow anymore. So then they called an ambulance, and I was taken to General Hospital in Minneapolis.

When I got there, they took me up in an elevator, and by that time I was really out of it. I heard these two guys talking, and they said, "I think she's dead." And I couldn't talk, so I couldn't tell them that I wasn't dead! Then I must have gone out completely because the next thing I remember was the next morning I woke up, and my mother and dad were standing over me with white smocks and masks over their faces. That was when they told me that I had polio.

Of course, my mother and father were devastated. They didn't expect me to live. My mom has told me that many times. She always tells me that! She's 97 years old, and still going strong. As far as the rest of my family, it seemed like they were all busy going their own ways, except for two of my brothers who were in the service. They came to visit me, and I really appreciated that.

There was a total of eight children in my family. None of the rest of the kids got polio from me. It was supposed to have been so contagious, yet I was home for a good two weeks before I went to the hospital, but nobody else got it. Of course, I'm glad for that, but if it was all that contagious, I can't help but wonder why I was the only one who caught it. It's almost like I was singled out for some reason.

Anyway, I don't know how long I was in General Hospital, but from there they took me to Sister Kenny Institute where they started my treatments with the hot packs. I couldn't swallow, so they didn't give me any medications. I don't remember much about the time I was at Sister Kenny. I think I just sort of lapsed in and out of consciousness. The type of polio I had, Bulbar polio, is where you can't breathe. You sort of suffocate yourself, so that's probably why I kept going unconscious.

I do know that I was only at Sister Kenny for maybe a couple of days, and then they took me to Sheltering Arms Hospital in St. Paul. I was put in isolation for about a week and a half, and then they put me in a ward. While I was in isolation, there was a lady who stopped outside the window there to talk to me. Her son had been in the same bed that I was in. She brought me a bottle of ginger ale and told me her son started swallowing when he tried to drink some ginger ale, but I couldn't drink it.

After I was out of isolation, they put me in a single room with a nurse who was on duty day and night. I had needles in my legs and needles in my arms, needles all over. I'm not sure what all the needles were for, but I sure remember having them. Finally, one day, the nurse who was taking care of me said, "I know you can swallow if you just try." So she brought a bottle of ginger ale, and I finally did manage to get a teaspoon of it down.

I still couldn't talk very well. I could maybe say a few words, but only in a monotone. I had no pitch left in my voice at all. My right arm and my right leg were also paralyzed for a while. That's the other kind of polio I had, and that's why I had the Sister Kenny treatment. They wrapped my right arm and leg in these huge hot packs made of wool. They kept them hot, very hot, and my arm and leg came back. I mean they recovered completely, and I had no weakness there at all. But, I had to learn to walk, talk, laugh, do virtually everything all over again.

I also remember being in a wheelchair at Sheltering Arms for a while. One time they set me outside in the chair where a ramp goes down across the street and into a cement wall. Well, I wasn't paying any attention, and all of a sudden that wheelchair started rolling, and it went right down that ramp, across the street, and into that cement wall! I didn't especially like that because the traffic was whizzing by.

I was lucky that I didn't get hurt, and after that they were a little more careful about where they put me in that chair!

I was there at Sheltering Arms until the 16th of August. Then they let me go home. By that time, I was able to walk a little bit and talk pretty well. The right side of my face was still paralyzed, and the only thing the doctors could think of to help with that was for me to stand in front of a mirror and practice whistling. Believe it or not, it helped!

When I was discharged, they warned me about going out and getting colds and stuff like that, and they told me to really take good care of myself. Well, the first thing I did was I begged my mother to let me go to a movie. We could walk from our house into Excelsior where there was a theater. We started out, and it began to rain, and of course, right away I caught a cold, so back in bed I went. I got so sick that I had to skip that whole year of school because I couldn't keep up with my studies. So I didn't start my junior year of high school until 1947, and I ended up graduating in 1949. I had no difficulty in school as far as learning. In fact, I was maybe even a good student. But I had to graduate a year late, so I ended up graduating with my younger brother, and that didn't sit right with me.

Later on in life, I met a guy, and we were thinking about getting married. However, I was kind of leery about having had polio and being able to have kids. So I took a trip back to Sheltering Arms and talked to the doctors there, and they said I shouldn't have any problems. And I don't think I did. I don't think the polio has caused me any serious health problems as an adult. I have had other illnesses though. I've had a heart attack, and I've had a quadruple bypass. I don't know if polio has anything to do with that, but I would think your whole body has some kind of reaction when you've had a disease like polio.

As far as other aspects of my adult life, I have one daughter who was born in 1952, and two grandchildren, both teenagers. I don't think there are any really serious effects from my polio, except for the fact that I choke when I try to eat dry things. People don't like to listen to me when I choke, especially my grandkids. So that's probably the biggest difficulty I have right now.

I really don't think anything good came from my having had polio. Maybe it's good that I'm alive! But I sure can't think of anything else, except that it has made me more careful about what I eat. I'm always being leery of what I eat so that I don't choke, and I'm pretty careful about my health in general.   I had a roommate up at Sheltering Arms. She had the same kind of polio I did. Like I said, we were warned before we left to take good care of ourselves. She didn't, and she had a relapse, so she's no longer with us. Maybe that's why I've always been so careful to keep myself as healthy as I can.

Marlene Krumrie

I developed polio in 1947 when I was 10 years old. I woke up one morning feeling very ill. I was so sick to my stomach that I was throwing up. I had a terribly stiff neck, and my back ached very badly. My mother was weeping and crying, saying, "Oh no! It can't be polio again!" She recognized immediately what was wrong with me because my father also had polio. He had spent a couple of years at Sheltering Arms Hospital after having been at Anchor Hospital in St. Paul. He ended up having such severe paralysis that he was in a wheelchair.

My mom called the doctor, and he came out to the house and examined me. I remember that he wanted me to tuck my chin down and touch it on my chest. I couldn't do it. In fact, I couldn't move my chin up and down at all. I was then rushed to Anchor Hospital in St. Paul where they did the spinal tap to confirm the diagnosis. The pain from that spinal tap was absolutely the worst I have ever experienced.

The polio was in my arms, legs, and back. So they wrapped my limbs in hot, wet woolen blankets. It was awful. The wet wool had a horrible smell to it.

I don't really remember getting other types of treatment, and I think that I only spent about two weeks in the hospital, so I must have had a very mild case. I remember the doctor telling my mom that I might have pain in my arms and legs later on in life. I do have some problems with bursitis in my arms, but I'm not sure if it's related to the polio. I've been very active over the years, and my arms have never really bothered me.

After I was released from the hospital, I basically just went on with my life. I didn't have any additional therapy, and I never needed to wear braces or have surgery. Actually, I think the fact that my father had polio had more of an impact on my childhood than my own case. I remember feeling sorry for myself a lot because my dad was in a wheelchair and couldn't walk places with me or do certain things with me. We had to get him in and out of bed, and my mom had to go to work, so it was my dad's illness that had the most effect on my childhood.

Like I said, I think I recovered completely. To this day, I don't really think that there are any adverse effects from my bout with polio.

Stuart Goldschen

I had polio when I was 10 years old, so it must have been in 1948. On the day that I started having symptoms, I remember that I went to a baseball game, which I didn't get to do very often. During the game, I started to get typical flu-like symptoms. I had an upset stomach, felt nauseous, and had a headache. I thought that I must've eaten too many hot dogs or something, but I felt ill enough that I ended up leaving before the end of the game.

Since I thought that I just had the flu, I expected the symptoms to quickly go away. However, they didn't. Instead, I just got worse. After a couple of days, we called the doctor. He came out, examined me, and decided that my condition was bad enough that I should be taken to the hospital. I was then taken to Children's Hospital in Los Angeles, which was near our home. They gave me a spinal tap, and I remember that as being very traumatic. It was painful and confining. They bent my back so they could work on my spine, and one guy was covering my mouth with his hand. I was terrified and thought that I was going to die from lack of oxygen. I think I hated the position and having my mouth covered more than the spinal tap itself.

The spinal tap must have confirmed the diagnosis because the next day they told me that I had polio. I didn't even know what that meant, but I could tell it was pretty serious. My parents seemed very concerned.

I spent about the next two months in the hospital, and I remember feeling lonely and afraid. I didn't understand my situation and what it was all about, and I had never been separated from my parents before. They visited me, of course, but they couldn't be there all the time, so I was essentially on my own.

As far as medical treatment, I remember getting daily hot packs for the whole time I was there. I also recall getting lowered into a pool and getting physical therapy in the water. I really enjoyed that because the water was warm, and it was very comfortable to be in there.

My back and legs were pretty severely affected, and it was thought that I'd never walk again on my own. I remember that towards the end of my hospital stay, they were going to fit me with permanent leg braces. When I heard about that, I immediately began to improve rapidly. Since there was no apparent medical explanation for my dramatic improvement, I think it was just the fear of having to wear those braces that caused me to get better. In fact, I improved so much that they decided I didn't need the braces, and shortly after that, I was released from the hospital.

After I got home, I slowly made my way to recovery. I don't recall having any therapy at home. I don't even think that I continued getting the hot pack treatments. Apparently, I didn't need them after I got home. However, one of the suggestions for my therapy was that I swim.

I was very lucky in that my father was a strong swimmer. He had done a lot of swimming in his younger days and had even worked as a swimming instructor at the YMCA, so he was eager to get me involved in swimming. I remember that he would have me get into the water and just kick back and forth for several laps at a time. I worked very hard in the pool and really strengthened my legs.

I remember that my dad took a great deal of pride in my progress and the fact that he had played a role in my recovery. He would often say, "Look at my son. Do you know that several years ago he had polio and couldn't walk?" That gave me a sense of pride as well.

I still enjoy swimming, and I'm a pretty good swimmer. However, over the last five or six years, I just haven't had the opportunity to swim as much as I would like.

I'm not sure if my improvement was due to my swimming, but I got progressively better and never regressed. I didn't need to have any surgeries, and in fact, I recovered almost completely. Therefore, I don't think that polio had too great an impact on my childhood. I did miss some school, of course, and I remember being a little nervous about going back. I also remember being the center of attention at school for a few days after I returned.

One thing that I do tend to associate with polio is a general lack of endurance. Though I've always been in pretty good shape, I get winded relatively easily during sports like basketball. I have always felt that I tired faster than most people, and I'm unable to get my "second wind" like many athletes do. Instead, I will work up to the point of exhaustion, and that's it. There's no reserve there. I'm not sure if that is polio-related or not.

More recently, I've been having some back problems. My back becomes quite painful, and sometimes I can hardly walk. It's mostly lower back pain, but not always. In the back of my mind, I'll sometimes think, "Geez, it's the polio that's doing this to me," but actually, it might not have anything to do with polio.

I've had doctors look at my back, and they can't tell me whether or not the pain is polio-related. I had a chiropractor x-ray my back, and he saw some problem with a vertebra that he thought might be causing my pain. He thought that if I saw him on a very frequent basis over the next three years or so, he might be able to help me, but I didn't go back to him. I would like to think that my back pain has a definite cause though, because then I might be able to find a solution for it.

Even if my back problems are due to polio, I realize that I've been a very fortunate polio survivor. I have no obvious handicaps, and in that sense I recovered completely. My brother is suffering from a very serious health problem, and he's been more or less living on the edge for the last 15 years. When I compare his problems to my polio, I realize how easily I got off.

I do think that having had polio has helped me to appreciate my own relatively good health. It's like many other experiences in life. If you've never been sick, you can't really appreciate being well.

Barb Grile

I was a very sickly child. I had pneumonia many times. More than once I had double pneumonia. I'm not sure if the pneumonia had anything to do with it, but I developed polio in 1947. I was seven years old at the time.

On the day that I was diagnosed, I remember feeling very sick. My parents called the doctor, and he came out to our house to examine me. I remember him holding my arms outstretched, and when he would let go, my arms would just fall. I couldn't hold them up by myself. The doctor called an ambulance, and when it came for me, I didn't want to go. They had to chase me around the table in order to put me on the stretcher. On the way to the hospital, I remember asking if the sirens were on. They told me that they weren't, and I was very disappointed. I thought that if I had to be taken to the hospital in an ambulance, they should at least have the sirens on!

When I got to the St. Cloud Hospital, I was put in a double room with another person. I don't know how long I was in that room, but it was a few days at least, and my mom would come and visit me every day. However, one day when she came to the hospital, I wasn't in that room anymore. Nobody could tell her where I was, and my mom was in a panic. Finally, she found out that I had been moved to the basement of the hospital where I was in isolation. She had to get permission from the doctor to come and see me, and before he would give that permission, he made my mom sign a statement that she wouldn't tell anyone I had polio.

I'm not sure why she had to sign that statement, but I guess there must have been a pretty big epidemic that year. Back then, everyone was afraid of polio, and so maybe if my mom had told other people, they would have panicked or something.

I must have been very sick, because they told my parents that I was probably going to die. I don't know why they would say that, but they did. My sister Donna also must have heard that I was probably going to die, so she gave me her doll. My mother had made us each a doll. Donna's was blue, and mine was some other color. I wanted the blue one, so Donna gave it to me. I suppose she thought that since I was going to die, she'd eventually get it back anyway, but I pulled through! I remember Donna being very upset because now I had both dolls.

I don't know how long I was in the hospital, but it seemed like a very long time. While I was there, I got the Sister Kenny treatment with the hot towels. I remember that they would roll in these big buckets full of hot towels, and they would take them out with sticks because they were too hot to handle.

At first, they would just put them on my left leg, and even though the towels were very hot, I could barely feel a thing. Then the polio criss-crossed to the other side, mainly to my right arm, so they started putting the towels on my right side as well.

I also got a lot of penicillin injections. I think I got a penicillin shot every four hours. I got those shots until my little butt was bumpy! I had so much penicillin that now I'm immune to it. If I get sick, and they give me penicillin, I'll just get sicker. So penicillin no longer works on me.

After I got out of the hospital, I don't think that I had any more therapy. I might have, but I don't recall any. I did stay home from school for quite a while, though. I think my mother was very concerned that I might have a relapse. I remember one time when we were riding in a cab and a police officer pulled us over and gave the cab driver a ticket. We had to sit in that cold cab a long time waiting for the cop to write out the ticket, and I did get sick after that. I remember being sick enough to have to stay in bed, so maybe my mom was right to be so cautious.

I didn't have much strength when I first got home from the hospital. But once I got my strength back, I went back to school. Though I think I was in the hospital a long time, I didn't have to repeat a grade or anything. I pretty much forgot about the whole thing and just went on with my life. I didn't go around telling everybody that I just had polio. I walked, jumped, carried on just like all the other kids. So I guess I more or less made a complete recovery.

I was fortunate in that I never had to have any surgeries or wear any braces because of my polio. Mother always said that the polio had settled in my heels and bunions, but I've never really noticed that. They say that polio always settles somewhere in your body.

I do have degenerative arthritis in my spine now. I'm not sure if that's a result of polio or not, but maybe the polio settled in my back. When I had x-rays taken, they showed that my spine is shaped like an "S," and the lowest two vertebrae are bone against bone. The next disk is almost gone, so pretty soon that will be three vertebrae that are just bone against bone. I did hurt my back snowmobiling a few years ago. It was kind of a jarring type of injury. So maybe that's at least part of the reason for back problems.

I took an early retirement from my job in 1994, and since then, my back has gotten much better. However, now I have some weakness in my legs, and I lose my balance sometimes. I can't help but think that these problems are probably due to my polio. I'd like to know what other people who had polio are experiencing. I thought that I had recovered completely from my bout with polio. It's just now that I'm starting to wonder. It doesn't seem possible that a person could make such a complete recovery from a disease and then have it start to bother her again more than 40 years later.

Chapter 10

Active Lives

Several of those we interviewed have led physically active, and in some cases, even athletic lives. The four individuals whose stories are included in this chapter have participated in sports and recreational activities that one might not think possible for polio survivors. While I make no claim of a cause and effect relationship, it is interesting to note that none of these four appears to be experiencing significant post-polio problems.

Dorrie Getchell

I am 65 years old. I was born in May of 1929 and had polio in 1930 or 1931. I was only one or two years old, so I am not sure of the exact date. That was not discussed a lot. Dates, times, and what happened, it's all rather vague in my family's history. Being members of the Christian Science Church, both my mother and my grandmother have had rather amazing healings, and I would say that my healing was also rather amazing.

As to my physical limitations, I have limited use of my left side, or more correctly, I have limited use of my left hand. I have very little digital dexterity with my left fingers, and my thumb is in a constantly closed position. My left ankle will not flex as much as the right, and my left arm does not operate with the same strength as my right. In fact, I am very limited in what I am able to lift. However, I've been very fortunate in that I have had no surgeries as result of my polio nor have I ever had to wear braces, use crutches, or a wheelchair.

I remember nothing about when I was diagnosed with polio, but I do remember the stories that my aunt tells. My father, or rather, my stepfather at that time, was a man who worked with horses. He had done a lot of work with injured horses, and that influenced the way he went about my treatment and therapy. I'm told that I was taken from my bed, put at the top of the stairs, and made to walk down the stairs, turn around, and then go back up. The driving forces behind this were my aunt, my stepfather, and rolled up newspapers! But as I said, I remember only what I was told.

I was never hospitalized because of my polio, not even during the acute illness, and I never saw a doctor for therapy or treatment. However, my grandmother ran a girls camp in Harrison, Maine, and I went to camp the following summer. I believe that trip provided me with a great opportunity for exercise and therapy. I was possibly the youngest person there, but after all, it was my grandmother's place, so my age really didn't matter.

My best therapy, of course, was swimming and hiking. I can't remember any specific stories, though. Nothing really stands out in my mind. However, I am sure I lived in the cottage with my grandmother and not in the tents with the rest of the campers.

I can't recall any definite impact polio had on my childhood. I think I was just made to act like the rest of the children with whom I was playing and associating. The only difference was that there were certain things that I could not do as well as they could. I was often helped with things in order to keep up with them. For instance, when we went up to my grandmother's place, I was not always the person to paddle the canoe when my turn came because I didn't have as much strength as other people. However, I did learn to paddle a canoe and still am able to paddle one today. In fact, I was a participant in many 100 mile, five-day canoe trips. Often, there were only two of us in the canoe. I paddled and paddled quite well. I was always on the right-hand side, though, pulling the paddle with my lower right hand and bracing the upper handle of the paddle with a straight arm and a straight elbow. Other people on the trips were very good about paddling on the left. They always understood that I had to paddle on the right.

On those trips we would always have to make the two-mile paddle from Harrison to Bridgeton, Maine. Then there was the two to three-mile hike from the shore of the lake up to Bridgeton to go shopping or to the movies, and I participated in this activity just like everyone else. I even played tennis. I threw up the ball with my left hand and hit it with the racquet in my right hand. I went to dancing classes, and I still enjoy dancing, even today. I did ballet, but I guess that my left arm was never in as correct a position as my right arm. I did archery; I did arts and crafts; I made jewelry, and I went sailing. I did all the things and took advantage of all the opportunities that were offered to me. Of course, I was better at some things than others, but polio never stopped me from doing the things I wanted to do.

Since I was never hospitalized, there were no polio-related expenses, and we were never involved with the March of Dimes or any other organizations. However, I'm sure that my polio did affect our family. Yet, it wasn't discussed a whole lot. I wasn't treated differently; I just couldn't always do things the way others did.

Polio has never really affected me as it might other people, possibly because of the way my parents and grandmother taught my sisters and my brother to react to me. I can remember no school or childhood incidents which were emotionally upsetting. I was made to feel that I was still able to do most things like others.

As for post-polio symptoms, I am and have been experiencing some minor problems. The problems basically are just an overall body ache and a sense of weakness. This is not only on the left side, but throughout my whole body. I visited with a very fine physician in Bangor, Maine, and he explained to me what post-polio syndrome is by first explaining about acute polio and how it affects your body. I know that in comparison to some people, my post-polio symptoms have been very minimal.

I also believe that because I have led such an active life, I have successfully handled polio's late effects by exercising and trying to be even more active. For instance, in 1980 when our daughter Heidi had to go to Jackson, Wyoming, she didn't want to take the bus. So my husband and I told her to take the car, and we would come and get it. We wanted to go on a long-distance bicycle trip anyway, and having to retrieve the car gave us the perfect opportunity to do so. We had been doing some touring in Scotland and around the state of Maine, but that trip to Wyoming was really a high point for me. We prepared by doing daily bicycle miles, and adding to the number of miles that we rode each day. I probably had accumulated about 500 miles before we ever left home.

When we started our trip, we rode 50 miles the first, second, and third days. From then on, we usually covered 65 miles, more or less, a day. On the first day of that trip my arm felt strong, but by the third day I felt a little sense of weakness, and on the fourth day as we started out, I really felt the arm collapsing on me. I took out the ace bandage that we had in our first aid kit and wrapped it around the elbow in a locked and open position. The day after that, I put the bandage on to start, but took it off probably three hours into the ride. Then after that, I started with the bandage laced around my elbow, but took it off after only an hour or so. Within a few days, I no longer needed it.

When we arrived in Jackson, we felt very downcast to have to get into a car and turn around and drive home. We had been gypsies and had camped out all the way from Maine to Wyoming. It was a great trip, but the reason I tell you this story is because after riding that distance, I felt like I could do things with my left arm and my left hand better than I ever could have previously done.

We enjoyed that trip so much that we said someday we were going to ride our bikes from Maine to the Pacific coast. That dream came true in 1984 when we decided to not only ride out there, but then to turn around and ride back, celebrating my 55th birthday enroute! This time we put in about 800 miles of conditioning before we started out. Again, we rode 50 miles a day for the first three days. After that, we averaged about 65 miles daily, more or less. We were on our bikes for five months, and only five of those nights were spent in a hotel. The rest were in our tent, here or there, but always in wonderfully comfortable situations. I came home from that trip from Maine to Seattle where I had seen the Puget Sound and the islands in Puget Sound, and I felt so strong in my left hand, and again, I was doing things that I hadn't been able to do before. So as you can see, exercise really seems to help me.

In 1988 my husband David started the Maine Island Trail, and time devoted to that project, as well as selling our home in Camden, moving to Appleton, and building a new house have minimized my biking. To me it's a personal loss, but I can't blame it on anything other than the fact that I have not put my own needs first. And now my hand is not working like it was before. I did do some weight training last January, February, and March (1994), and I felt a great benefit from it. I wish that I had the time to really get involved in it again. Why don't I do it now? Probably because I enjoy being outdoors much more than I enjoy working inside and doing that sort of thing. Why am I not biking? Well, I guess that I'm too wrapped up in other things like being a grandmother, working on an addition to our house, and being where other people need me. I know it's my own fault. However, I also know that gripping those handlebars for five months and peddling 65 miles a day did something for me. So I know there is something there that can be revived; it's just waiting there for me to get back on my bike or do something else one of these days that will revive it once again.

Another way that I exercise is by cross-country skiing. I never liked downhill skiing. In downhill skiing you have to keep you feet flat on the skis, which is difficult for me. So I cross-country ski instead. In cross-country skiing, you bring the sole of your foot off the ski as you stride forward. My non-flexing left ankle deals with this beautifully. I love cross-county skiing, and I do a lot of it.

We live in the country and in the hills, and I love climbing them. I enjoy skiing in those hills just as much as I love biking. I started cross-country skiing when it first became popular many years ago, but I had skis and poles that were too long for me. I tried to carry a left- handed pole, but after 10 minutes out, that pole would be dragging, and I couldn't carry it any longer. I never could plant it and use it as a pole is supposed to be used. I finally got shorter skis that had fish-scale tracks. Now I can climb with a pole that is suitable for me. In fact, I climb like a "madman!" My friends who climb and ski with me can't believe that I climb the way I do, even with my disability. But it's simply because I have a son who talks a lot about cross-country skiing, and he told me what to do and what not to do and how to climb in an upright position. He also told me how to correctly use my ski pole. However, using the ski pole in my right arm has subjected my right shoulder to a lot of compression, and I have had some problems. I know they're from using that ski pole, so I try to be a little judicious as far as where I ski and how much time I am out there. Nevertheless, sometimes I forget and overdo it because I am having such a good time. A little aspirin works wonders though, as does a little rest.

I think that some good has come from my having had polio. It has made me a much more sensitive person, not only to other people's physical disabilities, but possibly to any differences or challenges they might have. I feel I am a more sensitive person than many of my friends. I get less pleasure from talking about people's social, mental, or physical defects than many of my friends do.

Finally, I'd like to tell you about going to our local polio support group. At our meetings, we talk about our polio-related problems and how we deal with them. For many people, the best way seems to be through rest, recuperation, sometimes a nap, or sometimes a day in bed. Then they are well and back to their normal selves again. For me though, the best way has always been through exercise.

I was surprised to see two people at our meetings who I never knew had polio. One is a runner and a neighbor; the other is a friend, though not someone that I know very well. Both of those people moved through their lives with no outward manifestations of any physical limitations. To this day I see no physical difference in them, and I look at them and I say, "What is your polio problem?" Apparently, it is either hidden or just something that doesn't hold them back, but both are members of our group.

One of the things my husband and I did after our bicycle trip across the country and back in 1984 was to give several lectures about that trip. After my most recent visit to one of the polio meetings in Rockland, here in Maine, I read about the annual meeting at the Pine Tree Camp, and I thought, "I wonder if our trip is something that I should share with these people." I think I will follow through on that, and I hope that I have shared it with you in the context of how it benefited me. I also want you to know that bicycling is one of the most pleasant activities that I am able to do. I absolutely love riding my bike, whether it be six miles to town for a quart of milk and back, 27 miles for a day's conditioning, or just my few very favorite miles. Those favorite miles are my own personal LSD (long, slow, distance), and I know that riding those miles every day helps keep me going in spite of polio.

Dale Jacobson, D.D.S.

I developed polio in my very early childhood, so I don't remember many of the details. I think I had it in 1946 when I was two years old. It primarily affected my right leg from the knee down. I have some limitations in activities that require lateral kinds of movement. For instance, skiing is a little more difficult for me than I think it would be without my limitations. I really can't complain though. I have a successful career, and my disability has never really limited me that much.

Since I was so young at the time of my initial illness, my earliest memories related to polio are of going to the Mayo Clinic, probably for my first surgery which was performed when I was about four years old. I have some vague recollections of being in the hospital and going through some of the things involved with the surgery. I also remember having a cast put on my leg.

I had a total of three surgeries, and all were done at the Mayo Clinic, so there's some overlap there. My memories may run together a little bit. I do know that I had my first surgery at about age four, and my last one was done when I was in junior high school, either during seventh or eighth grade. There was another one in between there some place, but I'm not sure exactly when that one was done.

The surgeries were all on my legs and feet. I have always had limited use of my right foot, and in the last surgery, they tied some of the muscle and the ligaments together. At the time, I believe the procedure was called a triple arthrodesis. I think it was a relatively common polio surgery. The idea was to give that foot some more lift. Part of the surgery also involved fusing the big toe on that foot. It's now immobile.

My surgeries must have been successful because I didn't need to wear leg braces, except possibly for a short period of time when I was very young. Immediately after my first surgery, I do recall putting some kind of thing on my right leg, but I was so young then that I don't remember it very clearly. Later on, I do know that I had some special work done on a shoe in order to give me some support, and of course, I was on crutches at various times when I was wearing the leg casts and recovering from my three surgeries.

Because of my problems with my right leg, I remember as a child always feeling a little bit limited. Because of that, I think I really worked hard at athletics and other things so that I could be competitive. I didn't really ever view myself as being disabled, and yet there was always this feeling of trying to overcome because I knew I had a situation that required more effort on my part in order to be successful at some things. So having polio affected my competitiveness, and in many ways, that has probably been beneficial to me.

I was involved in sports a lot during my youth. I was lucky in that I lived in the small town of Zumbrota, Minnesota. Therefore, I went to a relatively small high school which gave me an opportunity to participate in interscholastic sports. I ended up being extremely active in high school sports. In fact, I earned a total of 12 letters for athletics.

I played football, baseball, basketball, and ran track. Though I was not a great athlete, I was the starting second baseman or shortstop on the baseball team all four years. I also was our team's high jumper in track. I was even captain of the baseball and basketball teams.

Because I didn't have any real limitations, I don't think polio affected my social interactions much. Actually, I think other people have generally been less aware of my disability than I am. In conversations I've had over the years, many times people have told me that they weren't aware that anything was wrong until they would see me in shorts and realize that I had a small right leg. However, I've never experienced any problems with social acceptance because of my leg. I think if my disability has had any effect, it was probably because of me and my self-consciousness rather than the reactions of other people.

I've continued to stay reasonably physically fit throughout my life. I play tennis and racquetball, and I've even won a couple of racquetball tournaments. I run two or three miles a day, and knowing that my right leg is weaker has probably given me added incentive to do that. I think running helps reassure me that everything's still working okay. Actually, I think that I'm in better shape now that I'm 50 than I was when I was 30.

I know that I've been very fortunate. I haven't had any problems with post-polio syndrome, at least none that I've noticed, nor have I had any back problems. Because my right leg is about three-fourths of an inch shorter, I know that back problems are a possibility for me, especially since I'm on my feet so much in my dental practice. That constant difference in the length of my legs could be a problem, particularly since I no longer wear lifts in my shoes. If I do start to develop some back problems, then I'll look into wearing a lift again.

As far as other effects of polio on my life, as I said earlier, I think that at least to some extent my competitive nature in athletics was influenced by polio and my disability. I also think that having had polio made me realize that I needed to pursue a career in which my physical limitations would not handicap me. I knew rather early on that my real calling would be somewhere in academics, and that was where I needed to put my efforts. That turned out to be an advantage for me because I focused on my studies at an early age and pursued a career that has allowed me to do the things for which I'm best suited. I think having polio made me develop a realistic perspective of what I needed to do in order to be successful. So in some ways, polio may have had a positive impact on my life and some of the choices I've made.

Even though polio has had only a minimal effect on me, I have sometimes thought about how things might have been different if I never would have had it. I especially used to think about my life without polio when I was in high school. I was fairly successful in high school sports, but I always wondered, "How fast would I have been if I had two good legs?" I think it's only natural for those sorts of things to cross a person's mind.

However, I don't really wish for my life to have been different. Although polio has been something I have had to contend with all my life, I know how extremely lucky I've been. My dad was a truck driver, and one of the secretaries at the trucking company where he worked had a very serious case of polio. She was in an iron lung and was very limited in what she was able to do. Thinking about her has always provided me with a contrast of what could have happened to me, and her experience has helped me to put my own disability into perspective.

Jim O'Meara

I had polio in the late summer of 1948. I was eight years old at the time, and we were living in the little town of Fonda, Iowa. I don't remember that much about the diagnosis itself. What I do remember is the night before I experienced what I always called "growing pains." They felt like cramps or a "charlie horse." I think most kids get them when they're young. But that night they were particularly bad, and I had them in both arms and legs. I remember crying because the pain from them was so intense, and there were so many of them.

The next day my parents took me to the doctor, and very quickly after that, though I don't really know how long after, I was put in the hospital in Sioux City, Iowa. I spent the next six weeks there.

I remember that I was put into a basement ward, and the only way anyone could visit me was to come to the basement window. It was a window like you would find in the basement of most homes now. The window was very small, about half a foot above ground, maybe 18 inches high by three feet wide with a screen. We would open it, and our folks and other visitors would come and talk to us through that window.

The polio ward consisted of two of those basement rooms. One room probably had about 20 people in it. There were maybe 10 in the other room, so altogether, there were about 30 of us in the polio ward. We weren't separated from each other, but we were kept isolated from the rest of the hospital.

As far as other things that I remember, I sure recall the hot packs.

They consisted of heavy pieces of wool cloth that they steamed very hot, and they would wrap those areas of our bodies that the polio affected with them. My left leg was affected. My right arm, my back, and my neck were also affected, but it was my left leg and right arm that were the worst. I wasn't even able to raise my right arm up to my mouth. That's how weak it was. The left leg was weak, but I could still walk on it, so it wasn't that bad.

I remember that some of the other people in that ward were in much worse shape. There were several who were in iron lungs, and I remember some who were very badly paralyzed. They couldn't perform even basic functions like going to the bathroom without help.

At any rate, as far as other types of treatment, we also had hot baths at the hospital, and I remember that they used **very hot** water. They would put us in a tub that was shaped like a three-leaf clover without the stem. It was a big stainless steel type of a tub, and I made regular visits to it. Besides that and the hot packs, I don't remember any other type of treatment. We may have gotten some sort of physical therapy, but I sure don't remember getting any.

I spent a total of six weeks in the hospital. Actually, it was six weeks and one day, but who was counting! And finally, after that six weeks and one day, they let me go home. When I left the hospital, I had a brace on my arm. It extended around my wrist, and the arm was immobile out to the point of my elbow. I could only move it horizontally. I didn't have any leg braces at that time. I guess I must have recuperated at home for a couple of weeks after I got out of the hospital and then I went back to school. At that time, I went to a one-room, country school, but that spring or late that winter, we moved, so I went to another bigger school. I probably would have flunked third grade in the country school, but when we moved, I got sort of a new start and was able to pick up from that point to the end of the school year. At that new school, I was treated like kind of an outcast. It was a relatively small school, maybe 12 or 14 in my grade, and I sure wasn't in the so called "in group" or the little clique that existed. I'm sure some of that was because I had polio and I was wearing the arm brace, but some of it probably just had to do with moving to a new school.

My physical abilities, or lack of them, probably also contributed to me not being in the "in group" at school. I remember that after I got out of the hospital, I just couldn't perform physically like I could before. I have four younger brothers, and they used to tease me and then take off running, and I couldn't catch them anymore. So I guess they figured that they were a lot safer! But in the long run, that may have been a good thing because my brother immediately younger than I am was always a terrible tease, and over time, I got so that I could catch all of them. The one next to me in age was the last one that I got to the point of being able to catch. It took me several years before I could, but I finally got so I could run just a hair faster than he could. So when he'd start teasing me and run off, I would take off after him. It would take me quite a while, but I'd eventually catch him. Also, if my brothers had problems with any other kids, they'd say, "I've got an older brother who will get after you if you bother me." So having those four brothers served as a pretty good source of motivation for me to get my strength back.

I remember that I used to fight a lot when I was a kid, and it wasn't all because of my younger brothers. I think I always had this sense within myself that it was important for me to know that I was a so called "tough kid." Somehow, I think that was an attempt on my part to compensate for the fact that I had lost some of my strength.

For a while after I got home, I made regular visits to the doctor, but I don't think I had any type of therapy program. I do remember that later on I had some exercises for my leg. I was supposed to wear the brace on my arm all the time, and my mother was very adamant about me wearing it. But when my brothers and I would go off and play, I'd just take the damned thing off and throw it on the ground. At school, I would normally leave it on in the classroom, but as soon as we'd go outside for recess, I'd take the damned thing off again. Actually, I think taking it off to play was probably more beneficial in the long run because it allowed me to exercise that arm and build up the muscles that weren't paralyzed. But I do remember that my mom used to get after me regularly about doing that!

I guess I must have worn that stupid brace on my arm for two or maybe three years. Then some time during the last year that I wore the arm brace, the doctor diagnosed weakness or some other type of problem with my leg, and so I ended up with a brace on my leg which extended from the hip all the way down to my foot. There was a bolt that went through the heel of the brace, and it held the foot and knee immobile so that it could only move up and down but not sideways. So, just about the time I was getting the brace off of my arm, I had to start wearing one on my leg, and I guess I wore that one for another four, possibly five years.

I probably wore some sort of brace until I was 13 or 14, and I remember that they wanted to do surgery on me too, but my mom wouldn't let them. I can vividly recall a visit to the doctor during which he proposed doing an operation on my right arm that would have basically bolted the arm to the shoulder bone. He wanted to just put a bolt through the bone in the arm and screw it into the shoulder which would have really limited my range of motion. It would have appeared like I had two usable arms when, in fact, one of them wouldn't have been usable at all. Well, my mom listened to what he wanted to do, and she just told him, "No way." Believe me; I've been forever thankful that she refused to let him do it because that arm is in relatively good shape now.

As a matter of fact, I'm right-handed which is probably a good thing because it caused me to use my right arm more. Since I used it for so many things, it really improved. My left arm is much stronger, so when I needed strength, I still could always use my left arm. But I play racquetball, and I play right-handed. And when I was a kid, I played baseball right-handed. Believe it or not, I was a pitcher, and one of my particular talents and advantages was my fastball. I could throw very hard which I think had to do more with the snap of the wrist rather than the strength of the arm because I don't have much of a bicep. My tricep is pretty well developed but not my bicep. Anyway, not only could I throw very hard, but I was also somewhat wild. That made the batters leery, so they would back away from the plate. I actually was a pretty successful pitcher in junior league baseball. In a six inning game, where there was a total of 18 outs, I once struck out 17 guys!

I've often wondered how good an athlete I might have been if I wouldn't have had polio. Maybe I could have been a professional baseball player. But, then again, I also sometimes wonder if maybe having polio actually made me a better ball player because of that drive that I had to compete.

I've also thought that I could have been a pretty good boxer if not for my polio. My dad used to box, and with five boys in the family, we all used to box. I had a hell of a left jab because my left arm was my strong arm. But I really didn't have much power in my right arm, and I'd always "telegraph" it coming. I've often wondered what I might have been able to do in terms of a knockout punch if my right arm was as strong as my left.

I guess what it comes down to is that I've just always wondered what it would be like to be physically whole. Since I had polio primarily in my right arm and left leg, my left arm and right leg developed even more than they otherwise would have. Those two limbs became really muscular, and I'm not a big man, but for my size I've always had a lot of muscle and good muscle tone. So I've often thought about what it would be like to be symmetrical and have two arms like my left arm and two legs like my right leg.

I think if my body was symmetrical, I would have had a very good build, because I did a lot of hard, physical work when I was a young man. For instance, we lived on a farm, and I used to do a lot of hay baling. I worked on the hay rack on the back of the baler and stacked the bales, which weighed anywhere from 80 to 125 pounds.

During the summers when I was going to college, I worked on a construction crew, and I did all sorts of heavy, manual labor. I also worked in a meat packing house as a beef loader. But I'd have to give my buddies at the packing house some credit there for helping me along because I sure didn't have the physical qualifications that some other guys had. I remember some really strong looking guys who came to work for this packing house, and they just couldn't hack it. But, like anything else, there's a technique to lifting those heavy sides of beef, and I had some real good friends working there. So when I started, they showed me the technique. Then I could do it, even though I was a much smaller person than a number of other guys I saw who simply couldn't do it. And I take pride in that. I still like to tell people that I was a beef loader at one time.

I really don't think that polio has had much of an effect on my adult life. It hasn't affected me in the sense that it prevented me from doing anything that I wanted to do. I played sports all my life: baseball, football, basketball. I wasn't that good at some of them, but I did play them. I'm not afraid to go to the Boundary Waters and canoe, though I am a little concerned about slipping, but I think everyone else is too. I do remember that one time someone asked me if I wanted to go downhill skiing, and I said that I didn't, and that was probably due to having had polio. But otherwise, it really hasn't limited me physically.

It may have affected me in almost the opposite way, and I've thought about this over the years. I think that it may have actually instilled in me a greater drive to do and be successful at whatever I chose to do. I think this is the result of people telling me that I couldn't do certain things so many times because I had polio. And my response then and now is, "Bull shit! I can do it." And mostly I did do it. So I think that I actually have a greater drive to succeed because I simply would not and do not accept someone telling me what I can and can't do.

As far as any negative effect of polio on my life, I suppose it has affected my self-pride more than anything else. My right arm is smaller than my left arm, and the difference in my left and right legs is even more obvious. I have no calf muscle at all in my one leg, and so I never wear shorts, just simply because I don't want to draw any attention to it. And I know that polio did affect my self-image when I was an adolescent and at the point of getting interested in girls. I think most of us are more self-conscious then about our physical appearance.

Otherwise though, I consider myself quite lucky to have come out of it as well as I did considering what I have seen with other people who had it. I have some limitations, but nothing drastic. I really don't think that I've had any of the post-polio problems that you read about, and if I did, I don't think I'd admit to having them. And I've certainly been successful in my career. After all, I've been teaching here at Saint John's for 19 years, and I'm currently Chair of the Accounting Department, so I must be doing something right.

Pat Zahler

I had polio in 1951 when I was 15 months old. Since I was so young, I remember nothing about the initial illness. However, my parents have told me that they realized something was wrong because suddenly I was dragging my left leg and having a difficult time walking. My parents called their family practice doctor, and he said to just observe me and let him know what happened. A couple of days later my mom and dad were in a panic and called again, so I was put in the St. Cloud Hospital. Since no one could figure out what was wrong with me, I was put in isolation, and my parents were not allowed to see me. After about three or four days, polio was diagnosed, and my mom says I went home shortly after that.

My mother remembers that she was frantic after I came home because she wasn't sure what to do for me. She wanted to keep me in a playpen so that I wouldn't fall, but the doctors at the hospital said I needed to learn to walk all over again. A public health nurse was coming out to the house, and finally, she's the one who said, "You are doing the absolute worst thing you can do for her. She's got to learn to walk, and if you don't let her out of that playpen, she never will walk again." My mother was concerned, of course, because she didn't want me to fall and get hurt, but the nurse told her, "That's how she's going to learn." So then things started changing, and before long, I was walking again.

I wore a brace on my left leg for about five years or until I was in first grade, which would have been 1957. That was the year that I had my first corrective surgery. I remember that I came to Gillette Children's Hospital in St. Paul, and I was there for about seven weeks. That amazes me. Now that I have children, I think about missing seven weeks of first grade, and I just can't imagine what that must have been like for a young child to be hospitalized for that long. When I think about my own children, I don't know how they would have kept up with their school work or remained in contact with their friends while they were in the hospital. The whole experience is just mind-boggling for me to think about.

As far as the surgery itself, what they did at that time was fuse a bone in my left ankle because I had very little control of my left foot. Before the surgery, it just sort of "flopped." There was not enough strength to allow me to step correctly, and if I picked my foot up, it flopped very loosely. So they fused the bone in order to stiffen my foot. Basically, it was "frozen," and it still is. After they fused the bone, I stopped wearing the brace, but I still needed to wear corrective shoes. I wore a shoe with the heel built up a little bit because my left leg is shorter.

When I was in sixth grade, which was 1962, I was back at Gillette Children's Hospital again for about another seven week stay. At that time, they did some more surgery on the fused bone, and they also put staples in my right knee. They inserted two stainless steel staples, one on either side of my knee, to basically stunt the growth of my right leg. That was done because my left leg was shorter and had pretty much stopped growing. That way my legs wouldn't be so out of proportion. I'm 42 years old now, and I still have two staples in my right knee!

After the surgeries, I had exercises that I needed to do. I remember doing leg stretches and leg lifts, those kinds of things. I think that I went back to Gillette every six months or so for a check-up and an evaluation. I believe that I went there every year through junior high school, so eighth grade was probably the last time I was seen there.

About that same time, I just sort of decided on my own to stop wearing built-up shoes. I couldn't find anything that looked good, and it just wasn't stylish to wear shoes like that when I got to high school, so I wouldn't do it anymore. Fortunately, that really hasn't given me a problem. I haven't developed back problems or anything, so I guess I've been really lucky. I was concerned that I might throw my body out of kilter because of the difference in the length of my legs. Not that there's a great difference. It's probably only a quarter to a half of an inch, so maybe that's not enough to cause me any problems.

One problem that I do have and that will be with me forever is that I wear two different size shoes, two full sizes different! Because of that, every time I buy a pair of shoes, I have to buy two pairs. There used to be an organization for people like me called the National Odd Shoe Exchange. Unfortunately, that doesn't exist anymore. I believe there is currently a new one that's located in California, but I don't know the name of it.

Through the Odd Shoe Exchange, I met a woman who lives in Royal Oaks, Michigan. She didn't have polio, but she was born with a cleft foot, and so we started exchanging shoes when I was about 12 or 13 years old. She's maybe 7 to 10 years older than I am, so sometimes it's a real problem because our styles are not the same. For all these years, she's the one with whom I've been exchanging shoes. I send my shoes to her, and if she can't wear them, I tell her to throw them away. If she can wear them, she reimburses me. She does the same thing for me. She sends me shoes that she has bought. However, I buy a lot of things that she just has no interest in, like cross-country ski boots and hiking boots. She just writes back and says, "Why would you send those to me? I don't have those interests." So I get stuck doing something that I just hate to do. I have to throw perfectly good shoes in the garbage because I just can't find anyone who could use them.

I did contact the National Odd Shoe Exchange in about 1990, and I listed all these unusual things that I had: hiking boots, tennis shoes, cross-country ski boots (two pairs), all these things that if anybody could use them in these sizes, I would gladly give them away. However, no one ever even responded. I never heard a word, so I finally just threw them in the garbage.

I did have kind of an arrangement with a shoe store in St. Cloud when I was growing up. I can't remember the name of it, but it wasn't part of a chain. It was just a small St. Cloud shoe store, and the guy there always gave me a discount when I came in. In fact, he's the one who put me in touch with the National Odd Shoe Exchange.

I don't have an arrangement like that anymore, so I just hate to buy shoes. I look for the correct sizes, and there are very few shoes made that come in as small a size as five anymore, so it's a big hassle. It takes a lot of time and a lot of energy, and some store clerks are not very courteous. They'll say, "Pardon me, two different sizes? But you'll have to buy two pairs of shoes." And I'll respond, "Well, very good; I'm glad you figured that out." A person just gets so tired of having to go through this same explanation every time she tries to buy a pair of shoes. People can be very dense sometimes. They'll say, "Well we can't do that." And I'll say, "Could you sell me two pairs of shoes?" "Well sure, we could do that." So I always dread buying shoes.

Now at least there are many self-service places, like Famous Footwear or Crown Shoes, and if I go some place like that I can be pretty anonymous, and it's not that big of a deal. But if I'm going to Dayton's or one of the other shoe stores, then I always have to explain to them that I need two different sizes, and they are very different sizes, five and seven. They kind of look at me funny, and it can be embarrassing. Never the less, I still try to get a discount every time I buy a pair of shoes. When I go in there and buy two pairs of identical shoes, a lot of times I'll say, "Are you going to give me a discount because I'm buying two?" They always just say, "Oh sorry, we don't do that." But I always figure it's worth a try. After all, if it's $50 for one pair of shoes and $100 for two pairs, they're making a pretty good profit. Anyway, that's my biggest problem from having polio. Buying shoes is a nightmare!

As far as the impact of polio on my childhood, I am the youngest of four, and of course, I had a life-threatening illness as a baby. As you can imagine, I could do no wrong. My brothers and my sister will tell you that I was spoiled rotten, always had my way, and was babied by my parents. I think it was not only being the youngest. I've taken some birth-order classes, and I think having a life-threatening illness coupled with being the baby of the family resulted in me being put on a pedestal. When my mom heard about this interview, she said that you probably should interview my siblings. You might learn more about what it was like living with me!

It's interesting, but my sister tells me that she used to be jealous every time I'd come home from the hospital. I'd come home with all these gifts and presents, all this great stuff that she never got. She's only 17 months older than I am, so we were close in age, and she remembers to this day some of the things I got. I don't even remember what they were, but she can describe some of the toys that I came home with down to the last detail of the color or the shape or whatever. Apparently, they were things that she would have loved to have had.

I think my illness was particularly hard on my mother. I believe it made her feel guilty for wherever this virus came from. After all, her baby was suddenly so sick, and I was such a baby, and they couldn't really do anything for me. I think that she felt terrible, and I think she really felt guilty. Not that she had done anything wrong, but I just think it was a weight that she kind of carried around.

My dad was probably more realistic about things and sort of a "let's get on with things" kind of a person. He decided that we'd make the best of the situation. He was just determined that there was not going to be anything I couldn't do. When I first started ice skating, he built a brace for my ice skate so that I would be able to skate. He was determined I would ride a bike; I would roller skate; I would do everything anybody else did. In fact, he said I'd probably do it better!

My mother was just the opposite. If I'd only grown up with my mother, I probably would have been over-protected and very coddled. I may not have ventured out and done a lot of the things that I've done in my life, because she tended to be very protective of me. That made my dad just all the more determined that I was not going to suffer or not be able to do things because of my polio. He told me that I could do just about anything, and that's kind of the way I've always felt about it. There really isn't anything that I cannot and have not done. We've gone on bike tours in the summer and have ridden 35 or 50 miles. The whole family cross-country skis. About the only thing I really don't do is run. My husband is a marathon runner, and he'd like me to run with him, but I don't enjoy running. I don't really think that it's because of the polio. I just can't get into it. Running is just not for me. As far as other things, however, I don't feel that I have any limitations. I realize that as I get older I might, but I don't now. I have never really allowed myself to feel that I had limitations at all.

I was fortunate in that I never got teased by the kids at school, even when I would come back after having been in the hospital. I do remember that during the sixth grade I came back wearing a cast, and I was on crutches. That was a very strange experience, but I had a lot of friends at school and in my neighborhood, and I was really never treated differently.

Back when I went to school, there weren't a lot of sports and things for girls, so I wasn't put in a situation where they were doing things that I couldn't do. I hung out in the neighborhood, climbed trees, and did whatever the other kids did. I think things might be different today. There are so many sports and other activities available for girls, and I probably would look a lot different than the other girls who were going out for those things.

One childhood experience that I particularly remember occurred when I was in sixth grade, and I was in the hospital for seven weeks because of my second surgery. When it came time to go home, I didn't want to leave the hospital! It's interesting, but when you are in a children's hospital, everyone there is just like you. I think that was the first time in my life that I was not a minority. Everyone had some kind of physical problem, and we were the best of friends. I even had a boyfriend in the hospital. In fact, the day I had surgery, my friends married us by proxy. They came into my room that night as I was barely awake, and said, "Guess what? We married you guys today! I stood in for you."

By the time I had to leave there, I didn't want to go, because those kids were my friends. I had so much comradery with them. My parents were, of course, just hysterical when they came to pick me up, and I said I'd rather stay there. I really didn't want to go. The other kids there had become my family, my friends, and I felt more comfortable, more alike with them as opposed to always being the one person who was a little bit different than everyone else. Even though I don't think people treated me differently, I was still always aware that I was just a little bit different.

That surgery in the sixth grade was the last medical procedure or treatment I received because of my polio. Therefore, I don't think that having polio affected me much in high school. Part of it is probably because I really never acted like or admitted to myself that I had a disability. I had a lot of friends, and I went to all the football games and all the school dances. I never missed a prom, so I don't really think it was a problem. There might have been some people who weren't comfortable around me, but I wasn't aware of that, and I think I did just fine.

I don't think polio has had much of an impact on my adult life either. I certainly wish I hadn't had it. It would be nice to have two normal legs and two feet that are the same size, but for the most part, it hasn't been a handicap or a drawback. We are a very active family, and I think I'm married to someone who's a lot like my dad. It never occurs to him that there may be something I can't do. He just goes on the assumption that we can do anything we want to do, and we usually do.

I went to college, graduated, and chose the career I wanted. I was a social worker for 14 years. Then I took five years off when our daughters were young. I just found a new job last year working in an elementary school, so I guess I don't see that polio has really held me back in any way. I do pretty much what I set out to do. I'm not saying that everything always falls my way, but I'm physically active, and I get out and do a lot of things.

My children and I have talked about my having had polio quite a bit. I don't think they really understand all of it. How do you get a virus that does that? They get a virus when they get a cold. Does this make any sense? It doesn't make much sense to them, but then it doesn't make sense to me either. They ask some questions now and then, but I think they are just trying to figure it out; this is something that doesn't make any sense, and why and how did it happen?

Putting my situation in perspective, I realize that I've been very fortunate. My biggest problem from polio is that I can't just go in and buy a pair of shoes. It always has to be an ordeal, and I'd sure much rather have two normal, symmetrical legs. However, I know things could have been much worse, and compared to many polio survivors, my problems are minimal.

Chapter 11

Late Effects

The five individuals whose stories appear in this chapter are all experiencing significant new disabilities due to polio's late effects, most commonly referred to as post-polio syndrome. Though many of those we interviewed are experiencing new pain or weakness, these five stories seem to best illustrate the onset and symptoms of the disorder, as well as the difficulties, both physical and psychological, faced by those who have it. It is interesting to note that these individuals had their acute illnesses at a variety of ages and had different degrees of disability after their recoveries.

Though post-polio syndrome is the common factor in these stories, there is much more to them. Therefore, as with the other stories, they are presented in their entirety.

James Frederick Berry, Ph.D.

I had polio in 1944 at the age of 16. I was left with weakness in a number of muscle groups, primarily in my legs.

The day that I came down with polio, my mother had put me to bed because I had a slight fever in addition to a sore and stiff neck and other muscle aches and pains. When I got up to go to the bathroom, my legs were weak and wobbly. I reached over to pick up a glass of water from a chair, and my right wrist and hand collapsed so that I dropped the glass. The doctor came to our house and made a diagnosis of polio. Since I knew nothing about this disease, I was relieved to have a diagnosis, but I had no concept of the seriousness of my illness. The words of a girl I knew from high school came back to haunt me. As a group of us were walking home from a dance, she had said, "What if one of us gets it (polio)?"

After the diagnosis, of course, I was put in the hospital. I was most depressed about the total isolation of the hospital ward. I saw nobody from morning to night except nurses in sterile caps, gowns, and masks. They were very kind, but I missed my peers and classmates. One bright spot was that I knew the intern in charge from the staff of the scout camp I had attended the year before. My window looked out on a porch, and my dad came to visit every night and talked to me. More than anything, I missed my dog. There was an older girl down the hall with a beautiful voice who sang the popular songs of the era ("I'll Be Seeing You" and "I'll Never Walk Alone"). Hearing those songs just made me feel sorrier for myself for lying there all alone.

When I finally got the company of a roommate, Chet, he was only there for a day, and then they wheeled him out to put him in an iron lung. I learned later that he had died. I almost sensed this ahead of time. We compared notes. We had in common that we had both been to scout camp that summer. He had played baseball the day before he had developed the symptoms. I had won an area diving meet the day before my symptoms appeared. After my release from the hospital, I found it very satisfying to visit Chet's mother. I saw her every six weeks or so.

The only break in the daily routine occurred twice a day when a physical therapist from the Lycoming County Crippled Children's Society came to do passive muscle exercises and muscle strength testing. She also taught the nurses how to do the exercises. She was such a sweet, gentle, and understanding person that I later named one of my daughters after her.

My mother joined the nursing staff in the isolation ward while I was there so that she could learn any procedures that she might have to do when I got home. I held the optimistic hope that I would get out of there and back home in time to start school that September. However, I was still in the hospital when school started. I later began to think that perhaps my former roommate, Chet, was lucky not having to face what was ahead for me. When I looked at my legs under the sheets, they looked like they belonged to some starving person from the third world. I had big knobby knees and no muscle. Once all the muscles spasms were gone, they finally let me go home.

When I got home, I was in a rented hospital bed in the dining room. The passive muscle exercises continued. The physical therapist came around to see me once a week. The first time she came, my mother was trying to get the dog off of the bed. The physical therapist made a fuss over the dog. That dog had always treated me as though I was her pup. There were, of course, periodic visits to the orthopedic clinic. After the first one, I was sent back for more hot packs and exercises. I did get assignments in English, German, and advanced algebra to do at home. I also had books to read. Most importantly, I got to see people again. The Scoutmaster and some of the troop members stopped in every Monday night. The Sea Scouts and the Skipper and Mate stopped in after their meetings on Thursday evenings. Eventually, I was allowed to walk into the living room, and later I was permitted to walk to the public library so that I could collect the information for my senior English theme, which was on "Polio," a subject with which I had first-hand experience, and to write a research paper on "Biochemical Changes in Brain and Muscle in Theiler's Marine Encephalitis" for the Westinghouse Science Talent Search.

During a visit to Johns Hopkins for a scholarship interview with the Director of Admissions, I took some time to visit Drs. David Bodian, Howard Howe, and Isabel Morgan at the Medical School. This group was doing fundamental research on polio. Dr. Morgan showed me how to do intracerebral inoculations into mice and how to isolate Theiler's virus.

I returned to school in December in order to take the exam for the Science Talent Search, and shortly after that, I was back at school on a regular basis. On the midyear exams, I got A's in algebra, English, and German. I made up trigonometry in the mornings before school and physics in the afternoon after school. When I was able to return to the YMCA, I lifted weights for strength, learned to make compensations in diving, and spent hours walking in the pool. I started walking at a depth where I was able to stand on my tiptoes with both feet and then walked to a depth where I was unable to stand on my toes. I also began running for stamina.

After I returned to school, I was physically exhausted, emotionally labile, and inclined to be emotionally dependent. Before polio, I had no trouble getting up in the morning, but now I found that I had to be awakened and forced to get up. This was partly related to the fact that I was doing homework until late every night and not getting as much sleep as I had before my illness. One day after a marginal oral performance in German, the teacher kept me after school. She commented that I used to be such a good student, and she couldn't understand what had happened to me. I pointed out that since she had already penalized me for being absent for 3 months by giving me a "B" for that period and that her "B"'s started with me and extended to a school board member's daughter who did "D" work, why should I waste effort working hard? I had other subjects to make up as well. I never could have told off a teacher like that before I had polio.

When I started going to dances again, I asked a girl to dance and she said, "Oh, are you able to dance?" I was so insulted, I just turned away and asked someone else. I remember that there was a girl in my class of whom I was terribly fond. After time spent talking with her, it was clear that my desire for her was hopeless, and I was heartbroken. Then I met the ex-girlfriend of one of my best friends. I'm not sure whether it was due to my illness and the related difficulties that I had in re-adjusting, but I tended to build up hopes for relationships that were far beyond reality. My expectations were so high that I was crushed when my feelings were not reciprocated in intensity by her. All my emotional eggs were in that basket. In the recesses at the back of my mind, I entertained the notion that these rejections were coming because I had polio. I began drowning my sorrows in alcohol, and after coming in late one night smelling of beer, my dad grounded me for a month. It was just as well. I had nothing to do but study, so I finally passed my exams in trigonometry and for the first semester of physics.

All the exercises I had done at the "Y" were really starting to pay off for me. One afternoon while I was running, the track coach timed me at 4:15 for the mile. He had also seen me high jump over 6'6" on a number of occasions. He asked me why I never came out for track. I told him that our gym teacher, an assistant football coach, insisted that only big boys made good athletes. Since I weighed barely more than 100 pounds, I figured I didn't qualify. I was becoming increasingly convinced that there were a lot of teachers who were ill-suited to their jobs. I had never been critical of teachers before my illness.

There was another girl in my class that came along, and this time the feelings were mutual. The relationship got to be quite serious, but it distracted me during my first quarter of college. I became so dependent and made such impossible demands that the relationship was over by Thanksgiving, and she was planning to marry the brother of one of the nurses I knew from my time in the isolation ward. I did graduate with my high school class in 1945. A high point was that I was presented the Bausch and Lomb Science Medal, and a close friend since seventh grade received the Rennsaleer Science Honor

Medal. These were the only science awards that were given.

I had a long-standing buried rage against my dad for hitting me every time I made a wisecrack or if I argued with him, particularly if he was angry or frustrated. I wrongly thought he might stop this after I had polio. I determined that if he did hit me again, I would kill him. We got into an argument about what I was going to do with my life. I thought I had made it clear for years that I was going to be a chemist. He and my mother wanted me to be a physician. As usual, he hit me during the argument. I swung from the toes and connected with his jaw followed by his nose. I ran his back into the sharp edge of the kitchen sink. The fight ended in a draw, but he never hit me again. He vowed he wouldn't support me in college, and he didn't speak to me for quite a while. As it turned out, I received two tuition-free scholarships, so I didn't need his support. I accepted the one at Johns Hopkins University since they got more research grant money than anyone else from the National Foundation for Infantile Paralysis.

As I turned 18 after I started college, I was obliged to register for the draft. Subsequently, I was called to take the draft board physical. I requested that the results be transferred to Lycoming County in Pennsylvania. The chief draft board physician for Lycoming County was our family physician who sent me to the hospital for polio in the first place. I wasn't surprised to be classified 4-F.

During college, my roommate and I used to double date with my cousin and a friend of hers. Fortunately, I avoided getting serious since I didn't have time for that. Though I had received an academic scholarship for college, I didn't do that well for the first year and a half. I flunked calculus, but I brought home two lacrosse sticks, and my dad taught me more about ball handling than the coaches. I played junior varsity lacrosse for the next three years. I also lettered in swimming as a diver and was a cheerleader. I enjoyed singing in the glee club for four years. I had to borrow interest-free half-tuition from the Lycoming County Crippled Children's Society for one year because I had lost my scholarship due to my low calculus grade. I was able to repeat calculus with a good teacher and got an "A." I began to catch on in my second year of college so that I got better grades with less effort. Accordingly, I got my full scholarship back.

When I considered graduate school after finishing a degree in chemistry at Johns Hopkins, the University of Rochester offered me a fellowship in biochemistry which I accepted. I couldn't afford to go to medical school, and I was not that interested in working with people at that time. Instead, I chose to do graduate work in biochemistry. Fortunately, I chose a research project in neurochemistry at a time when there were barely two dozen neurochemists in the world, and we all knew each other by first name. For postdoctoral work, I chose a lab where there was interest in the biochemistry of degenerating and regenerating peripheral nerves. Had I not had polio, I might not have had this interest. I am still interested in this area of study, and there are new directions I would take now if I were still actively engaged in research.

During my adult life, most people didn't know that I had polio. My wife has always kept telling me to stop when I got tired. The problem has always been that I was never aware of feeling tired until I reached total exhaustion. Dr. Richard Owen at Sister Kenny has always said that only weight-lifters, racehorses, and old polios run to total exhaustion.

I started having post-polio symptoms in 1968. The first thing I became aware of was a weakening of the legs and easier fatiguability. I noticed some slight leg weakness while climbing hills during a scout canoe trip to the Boundary Waters Wilderness Area. The second thing I noticed was around Christmas. We had bought a cabinet to house some of our stereo equipment. I had to lower the shelf for the turntable. I was lying on my back trying to screw in the mounts with the greatest difficulty. I had some residual triceps and deltoid weakness, but it seemed worse. I finally completed the task with my left hand. I consulted some of the neurologists in my department and had an EMG (electromyogram) and nerve conduction velocity done. Someone made the suggestion of amyotrophic lateral sclerosis (Lou Gehrig's disease), but even I know that ALS has a symmetrical distribution. Neck surgery was performed to relieve some spinal root compression, but the wait had been too long for reinnervation of the right biceps to occur. It seemed that the neurologists were out of their depth as they sought for diagnoses while ignoring my complaints about intensifying residual effects of polio. I went back to Dr. Richard Owen at Sister Kenny Institute. Dr. Owen had the quadriceps and hamstring functions of both legs evaluated by Cybex which revealed no quadriceps function but pretty good hamstring function. After eight weeks of carefully prescribed exercises, this was evaluated again, and there was no change. I started to use a cane for balance and to reinforce the weaker hamstring.

This weakness was very slowly progressive until sometimes my knees would buckle, and I would fall. I could not handle stairs without support or a railing. Up to five years ago, I could still raise myself up on my feet with the help of a six foot hickory stick. I can no longer do that. I have also slowly lost use of the extensors in my right hand. The symptoms first appeared about 24 years after polio and progressed for another 24 years. Initially, this was depressing. However, I went to several Sister Kenny-sponsored seminars on post-polio and found myself in a room with 200 or so people with similar or even worse experiences. It was then easier for me to accept my condition.

In spite of my current post-polio problems, in retrospect, the biggest difficulties that I experienced as a result of polio were the emotional lability and emotional dependence. I gradually got over these problems while recovering from alcoholism after 1975 through the help of the AA program. I believe these problems originated partly as a product of my age when polio struck.

If anything good came of my having had polio, it would be that it helped me to develop greater sensitivity for people with limitations. This was broadened in 1952 when I was teaching swimming lessons to fifth and sixth graders in Rochester, NY. I had one class composed of blind, deaf, or orthopedically handicapped children. I have worked in scouting directly with trainable mentally retarded individuals. I have never been uneasy or impatient in these circumstances. These have been satisfactions I wouldn't want to have missed.

I really don't fantasize about what my life would have been like if I wouldn't have had polio. However, if I had not had polio, I would have had the muscles to maintain a normal posture that would have prevented the bone spurs producing spinal compression and pain. I might have avoided three back surgery experiences. Of course, I wouldn't have the limitations imposed now by post-polio syndrome. I can accept all this, however, because I have never had any desire to trade the cross I bear for somebody else's.

Rosemary Marx

I am the third oldest of 10 children. We lived on a family farm near the central Minnesota town of St. Michael. My earliest childhood memories are not of life on our farm, however. Instead, they are of my experiences with polio in 1946. I was three and one-half years old at the time.

Apparently, I was sick for a few days before I was hospitalized.

My parents were very worried because I was falling and having trouble walking, so they took me to the family doctor. He was concerned about the possibility of polio, but didn't make a diagnosis that day. Instead, he sent me home with medication and had my parents bring me back the next day. It was then that I was sent to the University of Minnesota Hospital and following a spinal tap, I was diagnosed with "infantile paralysis with generalized involvement." My brother Jim was brought down the next day because he was having symptoms that were similar to mine. Fortunately, his spinal tap was negative, and he was sent home.

I don't have many memories from my time at the University Hospital, but I can clearly recall being in what I assume was an isolation ward. It was a large, glass-enclosed area that was filled with cribs. My parents were on the other side of the glass partition, and I remember being in one of those cribs, crying and screaming, trying to get out and reach them. My parents were standing there looking at me with tears in their eyes. I can only imagine how frightened they must have felt, wondering if and when I would be coming home.

I was hospitalized for a total of 10 1/2 weeks, though I spent only the first two of those weeks at the University Hospital. I was transferred to Gillette Hospital, where I remained for eight and a half weeks. I vividly remember the ambulance ride over there. In my memory, the ambulance seemed huge. There were several other children being transferred along with me. We were piled in there, two to a cot, with most of us crying. The attendant hollered at us to "shut up," but of course, that only made us cry all the more.

I remember only bits and pieces from my time at Gillette. I do recall getting the Sister Kenny treatment with the hot packs. They were very hot, and I would hate to see them come on the ward. To this day, I can't stand the smell of wet wool, though I never realized why until a year ago when we were talking about early polio memories in our support group. Even today, that smell, as well as the smell of some orange juices and bottled milk will take me back to my polio days. I also recall what I assume to have been physical therapy, though my memory isn't clear about it. I can see myself in this open area that seemed like a large box with bright lights. The adult who had me there stepped away from me, so it was almost like a setting in a photographer's studio. Several years ago, after reading my old records, I found that my treatment consisted of hot packs, physiotherapy, prophylaxis (aspirin for persistent fever), along with x-rays and photographs. I guess that explains the bright lights.

Other memories include being wheeled around in a big wooden wheelchair, though I don't recall ever being in braces. I also remember one particular visit with my parents. During that visit, my father and I played with a toy on a chain.

My mother has told me that the March of Dimes paid for my hospitalization. However, in order to be sure that we qualified financially for their help, my parents had to be interviewed. They were put in separate rooms and interviewed individually, apparently to be sure that they were being truthful. My mother didn't know if she should tell them about their finances, and she kept saying that she wanted her husband with her. The woman doing the interview was adamant that my mother give her the information, and finally said, "Look, if you don't want to answer these questions, then just take your crippled child home." That memory is still very vivid in my mother's mind.

After my 10 1/2 weeks in the hospital, I came back home. Although I have no memory of this, I'm told that I was very quiet, and apparently would tire easily -- something my mother would report several times during my early life. I was followed with clinic visits and was seen by a home health nurse. The closing summary in my records reads, "Patient was hospitalized for two months because of 'poliomyelitis.' She has done very well since discharge. The home is adequate, and there are no problems apparent at all. Medical Social Service Case is closed. 7-31-47."

Though I don't remember a lot about my clinic visits, one remains very vivid in my mind. While my mother was changing me into a hospital gown, I started screaming and holding onto her, pleading with her not to leave me there. I guess I thought that I would be separated from my family once again. Of course, my mother had no idea of the reason for my separation anxiety and the extreme homesickness which was to become a major problem for me throughout my childhood and adolescent years.

My homesickness prevented me from enjoying overnight visits with my friends and resulted in humiliation, embarrassment, and of course, teasing. When I was in the second grade, I started piano lessons. Because there was no bus service and the lesson occurred after school, I had to stay overnight with my grandparents, who lived in town. About four days before the lesson, I'd start to get weepy and become physically ill. I'd have stomach pain and so much anxiety that I would be distracted from my school work, and I wouldn't be able to concentrate on the lesson. The day after, I'd feel wonderful because I knew that I would be going home after school. I'd feel great for the next couple of days, and then it would start all over again. I was taken to the family doctor on several occasions, but he never found anything physically wrong with me. I had seven years of piano lessons, and although the overnight stays occurred only for a year or so, I believe that I absorbed only about three years worth of knowledge.

I never understood why I was the only one in my family who suffered from homesickness. However, when I was in my 30's, I was writing a short story about my polio days for our family newsletter, and I became aware of the separation anxiety issue which results from the hospitalization of young children and the impact this has throughout their lives. It certainly was a major issue for me until I was 18 years old.

Though I tired more easily than others, I didn't let that stop me from participating in childhood activities. I loved biking, swimming, playing softball, running, and horseback riding. I often competed with my siblings and other children, and there was always a drive in me to win, though I seldom did.

My left foot gave me a lot of problems during my childhood. I often side-stepped on it, and that caused quite a bit of pain. When I stood, I would raise my left hip in order to rest my left side. I realize now that when I rode our horse, I felt imbalanced in the saddle, but I kept riding anyway because I was doing something I loved. One time the doctor taped my foot in hopes of adding some support, but it didn't help much. In retrospect, I can see that I compensated a lot, yet back then I never gave the aftereffects of polio much thought.

When I was 12 years old, I was diagnosed with hypothyroidism because of fatigue and weight gain. Our doctor followed me closely for the five years that I took the thyroid medication. It did help, but in retrospect, I wonder if the fatigue was due to the polio rather than my thyroid. I've talked to other polio survivors who were also diagnosed with thyroid problems in their youth. Since my thyroid studies have been normal for many years, it does leave me wondering.

Because we were a large family and lived on a farm, there was always a lot of work to do. I enjoyed the outside work more than the housework. However, because I was the oldest daughter, I learned to cook, clean, bake, and take care of my younger brothers and sisters. Making and baking 10 to 12 loaves of bread every Saturday was just part of the workday. I also had my turn at milking the cows, barn chores, and some field work. My most favorite work was helping with the baling. It was heavy manual labor, but I really enjoyed it.

During high school, I was very active, particularly in music. My parents never had the opportunity to sing or play an instrument, but they provided all their children the with opportunity to do so. I played piano, played clarinet in the school band, and sang in choral and choir groups. I also sang in a small group called the "Michaelettes." There were seven of us, and we sang at school and community functions. We even appeared on television once.

My problems with endurance continued, however. When I started dating and going to dances, I seemed to tire more easily than the others. I was always glad to return home so I could sleep.

After graduating from high school in 1961, I decided that I wanted to get into the medical field. I considered becoming a doctor or a veterinarian, but at the time the long years of training didn't appeal to me. Since I had also thought of the nursing profession, all things considered, that seemed to be the best alternative. So that fall, I started nurse's training at the St. Cloud School of Nursing.

At that time, nursing programs were quite different than they are today. Back in those days, we not only had classes, but we also worked "split shifts." We worked in the morning, ate lunch, attended classes from one to four, then worked again until 7:00 P.M. Many times we also worked the 3:00 P.M. to 11:00 P.M. shift or the night shift. With the rigid study hours, we were very busy, but we learned a lot, and the school had a good reputation for graduating quality nurses.

I'm not sure if the long hours of study and work had anything to do with it, but I became ill during my freshman year. While I was home for Christmas break, I took care of a family that my parents knew. The mother had pneumonia, and her husband was unable to take time off from work to care for her and their young children. By the time I returned to school, I was exhausted and feeling ill myself. I was hospitalized for several days with a severe respiratory infection.

After I was released, I went back to my work and classes, but I still didn't feel well. I was later hospitalized in isolation with a staph infection. It took me a long time to recover, and my studies began to suffer. The Director of the school asked me to consider dropping out of the program, taking time to recover, and then starting over the following school year. However, I chose not to do that. I had little problem performing my nursing duties, but I remember having trouble concentrating on my studies. As I look back, I realize that was a problem throughout my school years. I always knew I had trouble with concentration, self-expression, and accepting criticism. I can't help but wonder if many of these problems were related to fatigue.

During the summer after my first year of nurses training, I received a letter informing me that I had been dropped from the program. I was angry and hurt, and I thought about enrolling in another program. However, there was a new Program Director at St. Cloud, and after meeting with her, I was allowed to come back and start over as a freshman. She also let me work for pay while I repeated my classes.

During nurse's training, I connected with music again. I taught myself to play the guitar and with four classmates, formed a singing group called the "MisChords." We sang popular folk songs and performed at a number of school functions. We appeared on television and played once at the Domino Club in St. Cloud. Music has always been a big part of my life.

I completed the nursing program in 1965, then worked one year as an RN at the St. Cloud Hospital. The following year, my classmate Jan and I went to the Bahamas as volunteer nurses to work in Bishop Hagerty's mission program. My responsibilities included public health nursing, school nursing, and some clinic nursing. I observed first-hand some of the unbelievable conditions among the poor as I walked around the island to see my patients. However, I loved working there, and I enjoyed our great group of volunteers. We all worked hard, but we also had time to enjoy our surroundings. The Bahamian people were wonderful and always seemed to appreciate our help.

Sometime during my stay, I went to a dentist for a check-up. I was diagnosed with a jaw infection, placed on IM Penicillin Streptomycin, and had a molar pulled. I developed a dry socket and had an allergic reaction to the antibiotic. Since I had been running a persistent low grade temperature, I was sent home to recuperate and rest. I spent a week in the hospital undergoing tests. While there, I found out there was no sign of a bone infection. There really didn't seem to be any explanation for my low grade temperature and fatigue. However, my Mantoux test had changed to positive, and since one of my patients was thought to have TB, I was placed on

INH for one year. A Mantoux test performed years later was negative, so I still have no idea what was happening to me at that time.

The day before I was to return to the Bahamas, I received word that two of my friends had drowned in a freak accident during a storm. My good friend and roommate Jan was one of the two. The hardest thing I ever had to do was represent our group at the funerals. Since Jan's body was never found, it was very difficult to realize she had died. After returning, I took over Jan's work as the clinic nurse at the general clinic. Jan and I both intended to return for another year, but after her death, I no longer wanted to remain in the Bahamas. There were over 20 of us in our group -- nurses, teachers, and parish workers. We were tight knit, close, caring friends, and the tragedy affected all of us deeply.

I returned to St. Cloud in 1967 and for several years was employed as a surgical nurse at the St. Cloud Hospital. My years in surgery were spent working long hours, and even though I really enjoyed my work, I was noticing that my problems with fatigue were worsening. I was also limping occasionally. However, I thought the long days were responsible, so I ignored my symptoms.

Because I was interested in surgery assisting, in 1975 I joined the St. Cloud Surgical Associates, which consisted of three general surgeons. As their RN assistant, I worked in the clinic, saw the patients with the surgeons, scheduled procedures, assisted in surgery, and joined the surgeons for hospital rounds and follow-through with the patients. I worked long days and numerous nights without consideration for my own health. During my off hours, I was downhill skiing, horseback riding, biking, and singing in a choral group. Though I enjoyed it all, I was burning the candle at both ends, and that was taking its toll.

In 1975 I had abdominal surgery for gallbladder disease. I experienced excruciating muscle spasms in my incision that necessitated the use of a narcotic just to have a dressing change. It took almost a year before I was comfortable lying on my side. My long recovery period following two later surgeries really surprised me. I was becoming more tired and more aware of muscle spasms. I stopped downhill skiing because of a bad fall that resulted in a sore leg and stiff neck. I was biking less, and I had fallen off horses twice within a few years, each time resulting in more injuries and additional pain. When I assisted in surgery, I was having generalized muscle pain, especially in my ribs, back, and left leg.

About seven or eight years ago, I started to have joint pain in my hands and feet. It was difficult to get out of bed in the morning because of the pain, and I found it painful to walk. Occasionally I would notice some swelling in my hands, but I thought that the double-gloving in surgery and the holding of retractors was causing some of the problem. I used to walk a lot and would frequently run up the six flights of stairs in the hospital. Gradually, I stopped doing that. My inactivity was creating a problem with weight gain which, of course, wasn't helping my joints and muscles.

In 1989, I went to Guatemala with a medical mission group from our hospital. We were gone 11 days and spent six of those days in a mountain village hospital giving medical care and performing surgery for those who had little access to health care. We worked 12 to 15 hours a day, and I felt driven to help as many as we could because we were there for such a short time. I limped the entire time. I wasn't sleeping well, and my back hurt. Someone found an unused back brace which I wore for most of the week. I was feeling totally exhausted, yet my denial didn't allow me to believe my difficulties were polio-related.

The following year I actually signed up to return. But by then, my sleep disturbance, pain, and weakness were worse. I would come home from the hospital, crawl to my couch, and rest until it was time to go to the clinic. I never seemed to catch up on my sleep. My left leg and back problems were increasing as were my poor concentration and memory loss. I was also noticing voice fatigue and swallowing problems.

In January of 1990 I saw a neurologist for diagnosis and, hopefully, a plan of treatment. I found her to be a caring, concerned, and kind physician. Although I was suspecting post-polio syndrome, she said she knew little about it, but if necessary, would refer me to the clinic of my choice. Following negative results of tests for multiple sclerosis and ALS, I was referred to Sister Kenny Institute for post-polio evaluation. Once again, I met a kind and caring physician. She confirmed that I did have post-polio syndrome and sent me to physical therapy for instruction in the use of a cane and to learn how to stretch my muscles. From there I saw a physiologist who tested my endurance level and set me up with an in-home exercise program that involved riding a stationary bicycle. However, I wasn't able to do the recommended two minutes on the bike. I have since found that pool therapy is the type of exercise that works the best for me.

Since my initial visit, I've been followed every two to three months by the Kenny Institute. Eventually, I was fitted with a leg brace. While both the cane and the brace helped, I was embarrassed to be seen with them. It made me feel like somehow I was failing. I was started on Mestinon to help with endurance and strength, but it increased my memory problems and actually exacerbated my difficulties with muscle weakness and fatigue. I found it difficult to drive my car.

In July of 1991, I took six months off from work. I wanted to rest, exercise, and continue with physical therapy. However, the time off didn't help, and I was noticing even more weakness and muscle spasms. My doctor at Sister Kenny was concerned about these additional muscle problems, so I was referred to a muscle and nerve specialist from the University. He completely ruled out the possibility of ALS and performed a muscle biopsy which revealed chronic myopathy associated with inflammatory joint disease in addition to the late effects of polio.

By this time, my life had changed dramatically. I was no longer able to work and had no choice but to formally resign and apply for Social Security benefits. I was denied benefits twice. In order to get my benefits, I had to hire an attorney and appear before a judge. That was a very stressful time for me. I was already feeling guilty about not working, and I was having a lot of pain. I felt like I had to beg for help. I first applied for benefits in March of 1992, had a hearing in November, and finally got approval in January of 1993. Though I was greatly relieved to get the benefits, the fact that I had a written document confirming that I was permanently disabled was very depressing for me. For the first time, I had a good cry.

Since my retirement, I have become more involved in my hobby of making pressed flower cards, and I've turned it into a small home business. The cards and flower frames I make are a means of self-expression and help me feel functional and useful. The first year after retiring, I tried displaying and selling my work at craft shows but found that to be physically exhausting. Now I sell through consignment shops and home sales.

I also keep busy with our post-polio support group. I initially went to a group in the Twin Cities, but because of the distance, I decided to get a group started in St. Cloud. The Central Minnesota Center for Independent Living Agency initially provided us with a facilitator, and I took over the leadership one year ago. We have a membership list of over 30, but generally about 10 people attend each meeting.

Our goal is to help each other and educate others. Post-polio syndrome is often misunderstood and not always accepted, but this is changing.

Currently, I wear two braces and walk with bilateral crutches. I'm learning to pace myself and rest more. I'm just beginning to accept the value of using a motorized cart for shopping, and I still feel self-conscious when using my wheelchair. However, it is getting easier for me.

The adjustment to my new situation certainly hasn't been an easy one. I always felt very fortunate to have initially recovered so well from polio. Now I know my recovery was a mixed blessing. The fact that I lived such a normal life for so many years has made the acceptance of my current disability even more difficult for me. However, I am blessed that I have a wonderful support network of family and friends. That support has helped me come to the point I am at today. I've lost some friends, but I have made many new ones.

In conclusion, I once read that when the never-ending problems and continued perplexities of illness get to me, God does not nag me about how faithless I am. Rather, He accepts my discouragement and patiently tends to my needs. I believe this with all my heart.

Jennifer Williams

I was born in 1947. In 1949, when I was two years old, I became quite ill. My parents tell me that they took me to the doctor, and he wasn't sure what I had. In my baby book it just says I had "Virus X." They knew it was a viral infection of some kind, but they thought it was maybe a type of flu. It wasn't until later when I stopped walking that they took me back to the doctor, and then I was diagnosed with polio.

I never had to wear braces or use crutches or anything. I just had to wear clunky shoes for stability. I remember my dad built a sand box because the doctors said that I should exercise, and my parents would make me walk through it bare footed. My dad also built a set of stairs, and he would take my hand and walk me up and down those stairs.

Other than that, I never really had any therapy, at least none that I remember, not until I was in junior high. I started having problems with my back at that time, and they started noticing that I had a slight curvature of the spine. I think that was in seventh or eighth grade, and I went to see a therapist once or twice a week for a period of about six months. I remember that I did leg and back exercises, and I had to do exercises for a while after that at home. I felt better afterwards, and I think that helped straighten up my back.

The only real problem I ever had when I was a child was that stairs were very difficult for me. I could only do them one at a time, and I always walked with a slight limp. My right foot and leg were always stronger. I guess my left side has always been my weak side. I'm starting to notice that more now with my post-polio problems.

One way that I was fortunate is that I had really good parents. Also, I was lucky to have a younger sister. I had to keep up with her, or I got left behind, and I sure wasn't going to let that happen. So that probably inspired me to keep going and keep trying.

I do remember having skinned elbows and hands all the time when I was little because I would fall a lot. I never knew when I was going to fall; I would just be walking along, and the next thing I knew, I'd be on the ground. I especially fell a lot when I'd rollerskate, but my sister had rollerskates, so I had to have them too. She had a bike, so of course, I had to have one, and I would get so tired from biking. I would make goals for myself, like I'm going to make it to the chicken farm before I rest, and then I'm going to make it to that tree before I stop again. I would say to myself, "I think I can; I think I can; I think I can;" just like *The Little Engine That Could*. And that would really help me, and then I'd say to myself, "I know I can; I know I can; I am; I am." That has kind of spilled over into my adult life. I just keep going, no matter what happens to me; I just roll with it and go on.

I remember that the biggest challenge for me when I was little was getting on the school bus. That first step up onto the bus seemed like a mile, and I just couldn't do it. For a while my mother came out, and it was so embarrassing because she would bring out this stool. But I couldn't stand the embarrassment, so my dad and the bus driver (his name was Bill, and I remember him vividly) got together and discussed how they could solve that problem. What my dad did was go out to where the bus stopped, and he dug a trench in the dirt. Bill would drive the front wheel of the bus down in that trench, and that would lower the step down to where it was really close to the ground. Then I could just get right on the bus with no problem. And nobody really noticed; nobody thought anything about it.

My dad had to go out there and dig that trench every fall because the highway department would come and fill it in. I think that he did it every year until I was a junior in high school when I started driving. We had the same bus driver all those years, and he would drive into that trench so that I could get on and off of the bus.

Even though my problems with the bus got solved, I think that starting school caused some other problems for me. The other kids in my neighborhood had grown up with me, so they knew my limitations, what I could and couldn't do. For instance, there was a corner market, and it took me longer to get there than the other kids, but they'd wait for me. Nobody seemed to mind. But when I got to school, I was in with a lot of other kids who didn't know about my handicap, and they weren't as tolerant of me. They used to tease me and say things like, "Hey gimpy, you walk like a duck." Even though it hurt my feelings, I think I just used to smile and not say anything, and then they didn't know what to do. I learned that if I didn't say anything back to them, they'd stop. At least that usually ended it. Also, I was lucky that I had a lot of kids who liked me, and they would go over to the ones who'd taunt me and say, "Leave her alone. She's nice." That helped a lot.

So I got through school pretty well. I couldn't do physical things, of course. I remember playing baseball in elementary school, and I would hit the ball, but somebody else would run the bases for me. And I was always the teacher's aide in the back of the room. I was smart in school, and maybe because I wasn't physically able, I became more of the book person. I enjoyed reading and other schoolwork, so I was often put in the back of the room to tutor some of the other kids. Sometimes I would even stay in at recess and study or help other kids with their school work.

I went to a private Methodist school from second grade through sixth, and that was because of an incident that happened in second grade. My teacher just couldn't relate to a child with a handicap. She was very hard on me, and I could never understand why because I didn't see myself as causing any problems. I guess maybe she didn't believe I really had a problem, so she would always say things like, "They're doing it, so you have to do it too. You know we can't play favorites." I remember one time when we were all standing in line to get on the bus, and she came up to me and grabbed me by the shoulder and shook me. I don't even remember what had happened to make her do that, but I always have had poor balance anyway, so I fell and hit my head against the wall. Of course, my mother came to the school to find out exactly what had happened, and as it turned out, the teacher was later fired. It bothers me to think that maybe I caused her to be fired because I don't know if the problem was her or me, but I do remember not liking her very much. And there weren't too many teachers that I didn't like.

That incident resulted in me being taken out of the public school and put in the private Methodist school. They were really kind to me there. That's where I started to do the tutoring with the younger kids, and I really enjoyed that.

When I got to junior high school, I was way ahead academically, so I went right into algebra. But the school was a lot bigger than my elementary school, and it was a lot harder for me socially. There were a lot of rough kids there, kids who had grown up in a lot tougher situations than I had. If they said anything to you, you didn't say anything back. So I got taunted and teased quite a bit, and I would just try to ignore it.

I remember one incident on the bus going home when this girl was taunting me. One of my best friends just went up to that girl and bloodied her nose. It seemed like the teasing stopped after that, and things went a lot better for me.

Because I didn't take P.E. in junior high, I was put in office practice and library practice. When I got to high school though, the state of California had passed a law that everybody had to take P.E. So instead of office or library practice, we were shoved into a room for what they called adaptive P.E. But it wasn't really P.E. We just sat in a room and did our homework. It was like a study hall. And the highest grade we could get in there was a "C." I hated that because it brought down my grade point average. So I was always struggling in other classes to get an "A" which would balance off my "C" in P.E. I remember asking why we couldn't do extra credit work or something to get a better grade in P.E., but the teacher would just say, "Well, I'm sorry, but the district office told us just to give you a 'C.' So just be quiet, and don't make waves."

I know that's all changed now, but back then, I don't think they really knew what to do with us. We were all just grouped together. There was everything from muscular dystrophy to broken arms, all in the same room. I think there were only two of us in the whole school who had polio, and we were just all put in this big room and told to do whatever we wanted.

Since I wasn't in braces and didn't have any surgeries, I don't think that my polio had any real big effect on my family. It was just that they had to keep me going, and I think that they were into that gung-ho. I don't think that they had to be with me more. It's just that every day they said you need to walk through this, or you need to do that, especially when I was little. Then as I got older it was, "Jenny, you can do that. If you can't, you can adapt to what you can do with it." And if I couldn't do something, then it was, "Well, there is something else you can do." They never wanted me to give up on anything.

I also think that they pushed me a lot into books. My mother was an avid reader; there were always books in the house, and she spent a lot of time with me. I learned to cook well. I don't know if this has anything to do with polio, but I did stay home more. Maybe I was just that person to begin with; I don't know, but I do know that my parents didn't treat me differently.

I remember that we built a pool; I think it was when I was in ninth grade. The doctor recommended that I have some water therapy, and it really helped. I loved the water. In there I was weightless, and I could do more things. I could hold my breath longer than anybody in the family, and I loved being under water. I still like water to this day. I even love the sound of running water.

As far as my adult life, beginning at about the age of 30, I have had difficult times. I didn't have problems before that. In fact, I had basically no limitations. I did have Cesarian sections with all four of my births, but that was mainly because the doctor didn't think I had the muscle strength in my abdomen to push and that I would tire too easily. Also, my hip bones didn't widen during my pregnancies, and the doctor was worried about that. He thought they would end up having to do a C section anyway, so he said we should just go ahead with the Cesarians.

I think it was about 10 or 12 years ago that I started to have a lot of back pain. I also started feeling fatigued more easily, and I was not able to do as much in a day as I normally did. And with four kids, believe me, I noticed when I couldn't do it. I would think to myself, "I did this last year." I could mop floors and vacuum and do all my housework in one day, and now I was having to take two days. I started thinking, "Today I will do the vacuuming, but I can't do the mopping because I would be too exhausted." I went to an orthopedic doctor, and he took x-rays, but there was no problem that he could see. I took in the old x-rays that I had from when I was young, and he told me there was no difference. He suggested that I should lose 10 pounds. Well, I wasn't that heavy then, and I had given birth to three babies already, and I probably weighed more with the babies than I did at that time. I felt better pregnant than I did then, so I knew something was wrong, but nobody would listen.

The doctors all knew that I had polio, but they didn't seem to think that my current problems were polio-related. They just kept telling me that I was getting older, and I would have to take this all in stride. "Remember; you're not 20 anymore." And this was when I was 30!

We moved to Utah in 1981, and it was a very different lifestyle there. We had a big garden and fruit trees, a bigger house, and the kids were older. There was more cleaning up and more yard work, and I seemed to be getting weaker and more fatigued every day. So, in 1985 or early 1986, I went to a general practitioner, and he looked at my history and said, "Let's send you to neurologist." Fortunately it was all covered by insurance, or I probably wouldn't have gone because I looked at his bill, and I couldn't believe what my insurance paid him for two visits. But he gave me an EMG, where they put electrodes in your muscles, and he said, "Oh, I can see that there is old polio here, but there is no sign of any new polio." I told him, "I know that. I have read all the literature, and I think that I have this post-polio syndrome." His response was, "Well, what's that?" He had never seen anyone with polio, let alone anyone with post-polio! I felt like I was his guinea pig. He had never seen it before, so he wanted to do all these tests, and that way if he saw it again, he'd know what it looked like. As it turned out, he couldn't tell me anything I didn't already know. I guess what really happened was I diagnosed myself.

He ended up sending me to a physical therapist. I went for eight sessions, and they put me on a very difficult regime of exercises as if I was recovering from an injury or something. And that wasn't what I needed. The therapist was saying, "Do it until you can't do it anymore. Do it until it hurts." Well, I did some reading, and I joined the Rocky Mountain post-polio group. They put out a newsletter, and I started reading stories people had written in and what doctors were finding out. I started thinking, "These exercises are all wrong." I needed exercises more like they give heart patients. I couldn't really do most of the exercises they had given me anyway. It was all I could do just to sit on the couch and do basic stuff to keep myself going. Finally, I just decided that the exercises weren't working, and I started to mistrust doctors and think that nobody really knew what to do to help me.

Eventually, I stopped doing the exercises, but I did have an exercise bike. I rode it as long as I could, and then I would stop before I would get too tired. I also had some weights for my arms, and I did exercises like they give to heart patients. I can still do my own house work, and I take care of the kids. I had to stop vacuuming, and that was mostly for my back. But I think there are many people with back problems who don't vacuum. So I don't feel that's a really big thing.

My problems did keep progressing though, and by 1987 I started to use a cane when I had to walk any distance. The event that really got me to start using the cane was when a friend came to visit me. She wanted to go to several museums and see some other things, and I said, "Well, that's a lot of walking. I don't know if I can handle it." She just picked the cane up and said, "Here's your cane." My husband had already bought it for me, but I wouldn't use it. It seemed like such a step backwards. I felt like I had worked so hard when I was little to be like everybody else that using the cane was going to be terrible. I thought that people would look at me more when I used a cane. I think everybody has a vain streak in them. You don't want people to stare at you. But my friend just made me go to the museum with her, and I think that really helped get me to use the cane because she said, "You know we are not going to sit around on our vacation; and you are coming along." Her strategy worked, and that's how I started using the cane.

In the last five years or so, I've been using a wheelchair. My house really isn't set up for a wheelchair, so I use the cane at home, and I have the furniture strategically located. That way I can sort of go from one thing to another and hold myself up by leaning on the couch or a chair. A walker would probably be better for me, but I haven't been able to bring myself to use one yet.

I've never been able to talk to anyone about this and tell them how I feel. My husband knows, though. He's having to face all this with me, and I don't want it to hurt him. But he doesn't feel burdened, and we talk about everything, the fears and everything else. He tells me not to worry about it, that he'll be here forever. I really love him for that. He keeps physically fit; he goes to a gym because he says he needs to keep fit so that he can take care of me. And I have four kids who are always saying, "Don't worry mom. One way or another, if you were left alone, one of us would take care of you." So I don't feel like I'll be alone and without anyone to take care of me. I'm glad to have a family that feels that way.

Also, everybody helps around the house. The boys have taken over the vacuuming and certain other chores. They gripe about it sometimes, but they're teenagers, so some griping is to be expected. It's interesting, but in some ways my disability is good for them. They don't see handicapped people the way their classmates do. Since they have a mother with a handicap, they're much more willing to talk to the handicapped kids at school. They even have lunch with them. I think it has spilled over to other areas, too. Even with minorities, they don't seem to have any prejudices.

But now that my kids are almost all grown up, I wonder what it will be like when they're gone and all living out on their own. I always thought that when my kids grew up, I'd go out and get a job. I did work part-time for a while, but with four kids at home, it just didn't feel right. So I chose to be an at-home mom. I figured that when my oldest got to high school, then I'd go out and get a job. But I never expected to get post-polio syndrome, and now here I am; my kids are grown, but I am not physically able to go to work. I can't drive, and living here in rural Paynesville, there's no place close by where I could get a job. We have one child in college and another who'll be in college soon, and we could really use the extra income, but I don't know what kind of job I could do. Anyplace that would hire me would have to be totally handicapped accessible, and I don't know of too many places around here like that.

So I have a lot of time on my hands. I've thought about writing, maybe doing children's books. I love to read, and I needle point and crochet. Those fill up my time. I cook, and I bake. I can still make bread. It takes me longer because kneading the dough is hard when you have limited use of your hands, and you're not very strong. But what I have found is that if I put the bowl in a drawer, it's lower, and that's what I need so that I can put my whole weight into it instead of just using my arms. So I've figured out a way to adapt.

I've been thinking a lot lately about the future of polio survivors, and it's my feeling that we are being lost. I believe we are a forgotten group; I really do. The March of Dimes was started for polio. That was the reason for it, and now it's gone into other things. It's not for polio anymore, but now we need help again, and there's nothing available. And this whole thing about the post-polio syndrome hasn't been publicized enough. There must be a lot of people out there who have it and don't even know it. They're dealing with their problems thinking that they're just getting older, and they may be going to doctors who don't know anything about post-polio. Everybody can't go to Sister Kenny Institute. Not everybody has a place like Sister Kenny in their area. There must be many people out there who just had mild cases of polio. Maybe they didn't even know they had it. Mine was so mild that if I didn't have other problems later, it wouldn't have been diagnosed. Then what would they say is wrong with me now? No one would know.

I think we polio survivors have a lot of fears. Where are we going to be 10 years from now? Is this going to get progressively worse? And nobody can really give us the answers. I'm lucky in that at least my lungs are healthy, and I don't have any problems breathing, but other people do, and they don't know where to turn.

What really bothers me is that besides the few articles that appeared in the newspapers about five years ago, there really hasn't been that much said about post-polio. There isn't any major campaign for it, no fund for it. Even Sister Kenny Institute isn't totally for polio patients anymore. I think there needs to be some place that is just for us, a place where we can go and get some help or at least some information. And what about people in other countries? There must be so many people in other countries who had polio and are suffering from problems like we have, and I'll bet there is nothing being done to help them.

In fact, not enough is being done anywhere. I know Sister Kenny Institute is doing a lot, more than anyplace else. And I know that there is a place in California that's doing some research, but what are they finding out? The information I have gotten recently still says the same thing it did five years ago. They still don't know why these things are happening to us. All they can do is speculate. Well, we are here, and we know something is wrong, and I think we deserve some answers. I think if we had an organization like the March of Dimes that was just for us, then maybe we'd get some answers. However, there's nothing like that, at least not that I'm aware of, so answers are hard to come by.

At this point though, I don't know what could be done to help me. My post-polio has progressed pretty far, but at least I have my husband and my family. I'm very thankful that my husband doesn't seem to mind pushing my wheelchair through a parking lot. I've thought about getting a handicapped parking sticker, but there are people a lot worse off than me. They don't have anybody to push them through the parking lot. So I think if I used the handicapped parking space I might feel guilty, and I shouldn't; should I? But I think we polio survivors do feel guilty because our parents told us we were just like everyone else, and if we wanted to do something, we could do it. It might be harder for us, but we could do it. I think we just got that in our brains, and it's hard for us to accept that we have limitations now, that there are things we can't do. Our parents told us, "You can do it; you can work around it; you're going to get better." But what I have now is not going to get worked around; it's not going to get better. In fact, it's probably going to get worse, and that's scary. But that's the way it is, and I'll just have to go on again and take a different course. Whatever happens, I'll just go on, because if you give up, then you might as well die. And I certainly am not ready for that.

Grace Audet

I had polio in 1952, the year of the big epidemic. I was diagnosed shortly before my eighth birthday. I remember some of it, but other things I don't really remember. My mom has told me that the day I was coming down with polio, I was out in my grandparents' orchard picking fruit. I guess I came up to my mom and said, "Do I have to pick any more?" She was sort of startled, because that wasn't like me at all. I remember feeling very weak, and so I went in the house to lie down. I remember telling my parents that I didn't have a sore throat, but rather that my throat just "hurt." I had recently gotten over a strep throat, so they thought I probably had strep again.

After a couple of days of those symptoms, I remember going to bed and waking up screaming, or at least trying to scream. I guess just a faint peep came out. I felt like the bed was turning over on top of me. I guess that was because the paralysis was developing, and it was somewhat uneven, making me feel like I was actually flipping over. I remember trying to hold onto the bed, but it still felt like I was spinning.

My parents called the doctor right away, and he told them to get me down to the hospital in Des Moines as fast as they could. That was quite a trip. My dad drove there at a speed of about 80 miles an hour, which was really unlike my dad. He was normally a pretty conservative driver. Just outside of Des Moines, we got pulled over by a police officer, and when my dad told him the situation, he drove ahead of us with his siren blaring. We drove through the city at about 45 miles an hour and went through red lights and everything until we got to the emergency entrance at the hospital.

From there on, my memory is a little hazy. I do remember getting curled into position to get the spinal tap, but then my memory goes blank until I woke up in the isolation ward. I remember being in an oxygen tent and having a tube in my nose which was hooked up to the water faucet to provide continuous suction. I guess one of the interns had figured out how to get continuous suction, because otherwise, they would have had to suction my throat out every five minutes or so to keep me from choking due to the fact that I couldn't swallow. My mom spent about eight hours a day with me at the hospital. She stayed in Des Moines with her sister, and she would come every day and read to me by the hour. I guess I was very restless, and the sound of her voice soothed me and helped me rest more easily. Many of the parents were only allowed to be there during the regular visiting hours, but they let my mom be with me as much as she could.

I believe that I was in the oxygen tent for 21 days. They actually thought that I might have to go into an iron lung, but I never totally lost my ability to breathe. They were also ready to do an emergency tracheotomy, but they didn't have to do that either. I stayed in isolation longer than most of the polio patients at that hospital, but I think that was because I couldn't swallow for the first 10 days I was there, and therefore, I couldn't eat. I think they were trying to build my strength back up before I went out to the larger polio ward.

After I got out of isolation, I was put in an eight-bed ward. And really, I remember the hospital as being a good place. Not that anyone wants to be in the hospital, but the staff there was very caring, and I have some nice memories of being in the playroom. The walls of the playroom had actually been decorated by some of the Disney artists, so there was a corner with Bambi and one with Snow White and the Seven Dwarfs. I usually played in Bambi's corner. That always seemed to be the friendliest to me. I liked to draw and cut and color, which always surprised the doctors and nurses, because my whole right side was paralyzed, and I was right-handed. I guess when they'd test my strength, I had hardly any grip strength in my right hand. But I still colored, and I still did my school lessons. In fact, I remember lying on my stomach under my hot packs and doing my school work.

I remember those hot packs very well. They used sort of a modified Sister Kenny method at that hospital. There were only a few therapists who were actually trained in the Kenny method, but all the therapists used the hot packs. I think that was just standard procedure for that hospital, but some therapists also used more traditional methods. I think they probably just tended to use whatever seemed to work for the particular patient with whom they were working at the time.

I also remember getting penicillin shots twice a day while I was in isolation. They did that to help arrest the infection and to get me through the critical stage of the disease. I have no idea if the penicillin actually helped.

I spent a total of 79 days in the hospital. When I came home, I still had a lot of muscle weakness, mostly in my upper body, particularly my trunk and neck. I had a rather strenuous exercise program that I had to do at home. It took about three and a half hours to do all of my exercises. I remember that my dad rigged up a library table with an overhead framework with pulleys and ropes, so I could do weight lifting with all of my muscle groups. I did most of them with my right side since that was where I had the major paralysis. I did a few with my left leg, and I remember doing a lot of sit-ups, stretches, and back extensions. I guess it took about six months of doing those exercises before I was able to raise my right arm.

After I returned to school full time, my exercise schedule was cut down to about two and a half hours a day. With school, my exercises, and farm chores, I didn't really have the time or energy to do much else. Because of that, I think I never really learned how to play, or if I did know how to play before I had polio, I forgot how. It's interesting, but I never really realized that until I had my own children. I remember when our oldest was two years old, he looked at me one day and said, "Mommy, you don't know how to play; do you?" And then it hit me. All those years when I was doing those exercises, which was basically from age 10 to 12, I didn't have time to play, and on those rare occasions when I did have the time, I didn't have the energy. I guess that reading became my play. I read, did puzzles, handicrafts, but I never did the things that normal children do like getting out and playing ball or running. I could see that my son was right; I really didn't know how to play. I had to learn that as an adult so I could play with my children.

At any rate, after a couple of years of doing those exercises, I was basically told that I could do whatever I wanted. And what I wanted to do was play in the band. I tried to play a wind instrument, but I kept getting ear infections. Because of weakness in my throat muscles from polio, I apparently couldn't close off the passages to my ears when I had a cold or something. I tried the drums, and I was doing fairly well. However, then I played the cymbals for two days in concert band, and I got muscle spasms under my shoulder blade because apparently those muscles were also weak. So, unfortunately,

I had to give that up.

Eventually we moved to Tucson, and there was quite a change in lifestyle. We weren't living on a farm anymore, so we didn't have all the chores to do, and we no longer had a garden. The Arizona heat and sunshine also represented quite a change, and I started to feel a lot better. I even started walking the mile or so to school everyday, and I think that exercise helped me as well. In fact, after we had lived there for about a year, I was able to go off of all pain medication. For the previous couple of years, I had been taking as many as 12 or 16 aspirins a day, which was an awfully high dosage for a high school freshman or sophomore.

I was even able to start taking P.E. again. At first, I was in modified P.E. That class was in the room next to the modern dance class, and I remember looking in the dance room and thinking, "Gee, they're doing a lot of stretches and other things that I think I could do. Maybe I should try that." So we talked to the instructor, and she said she'd be glad to let me try her class, and if there was something I couldn't do, I should just let her know. I tried the dance class and did pretty well, but there were some things I couldn't do, and a lot of times I only learned I shouldn't do them after the fact. For instance, there was an exercise that involved raising your head up off of the floor and then shifting your legs. Well, after doing that for a couple of days, I couldn't stop coughing. I just didn't have the neck muscles to allow me to do that, and so I wasn't strengthening the muscles. Rather, I was damaging them through overuse. I've really been battling that sort of thing all of my life. I just didn't want to accept the fact that there were so many things I couldn't do. However, I had no choice but to drop a lot of things when I realized they were things that might be harmful for me.

After I finished high school, I went to the University of Arizona where I had a full scholarship. I felt so good while I was there that I think my whole personality changed. I was actually nicknamed "Bubbles" by some of the people at the Methodist Student Center because I seemed so happy all the time. I remember asking my mom if I was ever like that before, and she told me that's the way I was before I had polio.

Unfortunately, I ended up spending only two years at the University of Arizona. I wanted to go into occupational therapy, and in order to do that, I had to transfer to another university. I remember that my first choice was Texas Women's College, but I was advised that I needed more social interaction, and that a women's college wouldn't meet my needs. Instead, I ended up transferring to the University of Iowa. Unfortunately, those cold, damp Iowa winters began taking their toll on me, but by then, I had already met my husband who was a student instructor at Iowa, so I stayed there. He was a northern boy, born in Canada and raised in Milwaukee, and though I took him out to Arizona, he preferred living in the North. After we got married, of course, I had to go wherever he went. He became a minister, and the church found him a parish in Wisconsin.

As it turned out, I didn't go into occupational therapy after all. Instead, I got a teaching degree, and I ended up getting a job teaching kindergarten that first year after college, but by Thanksgiving, I was so fatigued that I just couldn't handle it anymore. I loved the kids and the teaching. In fact, I would have paid them to let me teach, but I had developed what is called "fatigue-induced depression," though I didn't realize that's what I had until years later, and I just couldn't continue. I really wanted to be able to teach, so it was very frustrating for me, but I just saw that I was unable to do it full time. Therefore, I requested a termination of my contract in January.

There was a young woman in town who had finished her teaching degree in January and desperately needed work because her husband had become ill. Fortunately, she was an excellent teacher. I felt very good about her getting the job. It was almost like I had been a space holder for her, so I guess something good came of that situation.

Since then, I've occasionally done substitute teaching. I can substitute for three or four days at a time and enjoy it, but I couldn't do it for three or four weeks in a row. It would just wear me down. So for the most part, I've worked at home with our ministries, and I've enjoyed that very much. I've also been a mom and a homemaker.

I was blessed that all of our children were relatively easy babies to take care of. I think it would have been very difficult for me if I would have had fussy or strong-willed children. I don't know if I would have had the energy because I guess that I've had the sort of fatigue problems throughout my adult life that a lot of post-polio patients develop. It took me a lot of years to admit that to myself, but I finally came to grips with the fact that my fatigue was polio-related. I can remember talking to our family physician when I was pregnant with Sara, who's 14 now, and telling him, "I'm sick and tired of being sick and tired!" I guess I was about 33 or 34 then, and I was trying to do all the things that I remember my mother doing, but I just couldn't keep up. I could do most everything, but I'd get muscle spasms, and I would get so run-down that I was having bronchial infections every fall. I'd start coughing and coughing because I was having muscle spasms in my throat. And I'd think, "Why can't I keep going?" People would ask me how I was doing, and I'd say, "Well, it only hurts when I laugh, talk, or breathe!" I never realized that when the muscles you breathe with are affected, everything that you do increases the need for oxygen, and if your breathing can't supply enough oxygen, then you just can't keep going.

I guess I really figured out that I had post-polio syndrome shortly before we moved here to Becker which was about six years ago. At that time, my husband had suggested that perhaps my low energy was a result of not getting enough exercise. So I went to a sports and health club and tried working out. Walking on the smooth track and stretching helped, but a lot of the things I tried to do, particularly the upper body things, just made me worse. About that same time, my mother sent me an article about post-polio syndrome because she was quite concerned about the state I was getting myself into. I made an appointment with my doctor in St. Cloud and asked him if he knew anything about post-polio problems. He said that he was just beginning to learn about them, so he referred me to a neurologist in the Twin Cities who he thought could help me. I saw him a few times, and he told me that I probably did have post-polio syndrome.

It's interesting, but the diagnosis almost came as a relief to me. When you look as healthy as I looked, there's a tendency for people to think that this is all in your head, that you're a hypochondriac. When a physician acknowledges that this is real and that you're working with a very compromised neurological system, you feel a sense of relief. Also, once you know what the problem is, then you can start to figure out what to do about it. With the help of the neurologist, that's what I did.

I started going to a physical therapist in Monticello, and though he said he didn't have all the answers, he thought that he could do some things to help. Outside of just gently suggesting that I cut down on my activities a bit, he started to do some therapy with me. The therapy was mostly for relief of my muscle spasms and consisted of ultrasound and massage. The therapy really helped, but I have also learned which activities are particularly harmful for my body. When I reduced the number of those really stressful activities, I found that I was much more able to think clearly and do things in ways that aren't so exhausting.

About three or four years ago, I started wearing a leg brace, and it's helped a lot in giving me confidence when I walk. I'm not nearly as afraid of falling as I was before I wore the brace. I really didn't have too hard a time accepting the brace because it felt so good to be able to walk again without the fear of tripping over my own feet. I know that some people have problems accepting the fact that they have to wear a brace, but for me it helped my functioning so much that I found myself wishing that I had started wearing the brace years ago. I think that a lot of people remember how heavy and ugly the old metal braces were, but the new ones are completely different.

I'm taking a medication called Mestinon which helps my muscles work a little better. Dr. Owen from Sister Kenny Institute prescribed that. He has had polio too, so he can really understand what I'm experiencing. Talking to him has also helped me to understand what is happening to my body. I understand now that those of us who have had polio don't feel fatigue the same way a person with a normal body does. People with an undamaged neurological system will feel fatigued when they have used about two-thirds of their muscle capacity. So even though they feel fatigued, they still have some strength in reserve. But when those of us who had polio feel exhausted, we have often already used up all of our muscle reserve. If we try to go beyond that point, then we are doing damage that we'll pay for later with pain or possibly even loss of function. In the past, I've tended to overuse my muscles and work to complete exhaustion. Now, I'm trying to learn what my limits are and not go past them. I have a handicapped parking sticker, and that's really great when there's ice in a parking lot. I've finally been able to accept the fact that I need it, but I still only use it when I absolutely have to.

Another thing that I've found helpful is being a part of a post-polio support group. I actually helped start the support group here in St. Cloud. I had originally tried to make connections with one in the Twin Cities, but it's too long a drive for me. Thirty or 40 miles is about the maximum that I can drive.

Over the years, I have, of course, thought about the things I might have done or would like to have done if I wouldn't have had polio. Two things that I've thought about are being a dancer and playing the violin. I did get sort of a taste of dance when I took the modern dance class in high school, and I really enjoyed it. I know it's unlikely that I ever could have been a professional dancer, rather I just wish I could have done more dancing and taken more dance classes. Though I've never played the violin, I love the instrument, and I wish I had the strength in my neck and arms to allow me to play it.

I've learned not to dwell on those things that I can't do, though. In fact, I have been seeing a psychologist who has helped me accept the realities of my physical limitations. In one sense, a part of me could acknowledge that those limits were there, but then there was another part of me thinking that my condition was something to try and overcome instead of something that I needed to learn to live with. However, I'm learning now that my limits, my boundaries, are like a picture frame. If I live within those boundaries, my life can be like a well-framed picture, and that picture can be filled with beauty and joy. I can do lots of things that fit within that picture frame, but if I try to do too much, then it all spills out and ruins the most important things, the beauty and joy that I've put in the center of the picture. So I learned that I was trying to stretch my limits instead of accepting them, and I've also learned that accepting those limits helps me to see the possibilities within those limits.

It's not a matter of just being resigned to the things that I can't do. It's also a matter of discovering and then doing the things that I can do. And now that I've come to that point of acceptance, I'm feeling like I'm about ready to terminate my work with the psychologist and just get on with doing those things that I can do and enjoy doing.

Janice Johnson Gradin

The summer of 1956 was a very busy time for me. I was 15 years old and finishing my first year of high school. I had final exams at school, confirmation, and my brother got married that June. I was involved in church activities and was baby-sitting a lot. I often felt tired, and I experienced some fainting spells. My parents wouldn't let me go to the county fair because there were "too many polio germs" there. I recall being very upset about that.

That year was also about the time that the Salk vaccine was developed. However, a lot of people from my home town of Evansville, Minnesota didn't get vaccinated and wouldn't take their children to be vaccinated. They didn't know if the vaccine was safe and were afraid that they might actually catch polio from the vaccine.

I didn't get vaccinated, and on August eighth of that year, I came down with polio. It was a very hot day, and I remember feeling like I had the flu. I was supposed to help my dad mow the lawn. He had just gotten a new lawn mower, but I told him that I didn't feel well.

He said, "Well then, just go take a nap." I did, and it seemed as though my whole body just gave in to the polio virus. I became very sick. My neck was stiff; my head ached; and I had a very sore throat. I developed a high temperature and became very weak.

The next day my parents called the doctor, and he came out to the house and gave me some sulfa pills for my fever. He told my parents that if I wasn't any better by Friday he wanted me to go to the hospital for tests. Well, Friday came, and I still wasn't any better. So mom and I rode to the hospital in Alexandria. They gave me a spinal tap, and it showed that I had polio.

I was put in isolation for a week. It was a very scary and lonesome time for me. I was very sick and hurt all over. I fell down if I tried to get out of bed and walk. I couldn't have any visitors except my mom, and she could only stay for five minutes. I did get a lot of cards and letters though, and they helped keep my spirits up.

When the people in the Evansville area found out that I had polio, they changed their minds about the vaccine. Suddenly, long lines formed in front of the clinic so that everyone could get their shots. I guess my illness really woke up the town.

Now that people knew that I had polio, some were afraid to even buy groceries in the same store where my parents shopped. Some wouldn't even walk on the same side of the street as my parents. They were afraid they might catch polio from them. For the most part though, people were very kind. Many sent cards and gifts and prayed for me.

This was, of course, a very difficult time for my family. They wondered how much damage the polio virus had done to me and how long it would take for me to recover, or if I would ever recover. I had a young niece and nephew, and the family was worried that they would get polio too. We were all very thankful that they didn't.

One week after I went into the hospital, my mom, dad, and the doctor came into my room. I remember being very scared of what was coming next. They had decided that I should be transferred to Sister Kenny Institute in Minneapolis because that was where polio patients could get the best care. That was my first trip to Minneapolis. It seemed so far away back in those days. They put me in an ambulance first thing the next morning, and the trip took most of the day. When we got to the Minneapolis city limits, they turned on the lights and the siren. It was a very frightening experience.

I arrived at Sister Kenny Institute some time that afternoon. I remember it was a Saturday. I was very weak and hurt all over, so one of the nurses aides started up the "cooker" and heated up a hot pack to put on me. When she put it on, it was very hot (140 degrees), and I started to scream. She meant well but hadn't explained what it would feel like after she wrapped me in it.

Those first couple of days at Sister Kenny were very scary for me. I was there all by myself. My parents were 160 miles away. I had never been away from home before, and I didn't know what was going to happen next.

On Monday, the doctors and therapists checked me over. My doctor from Alexandria hadn't sent enough information about my spinal tap, so they had to do it over again. I had to lie flat in bed for eight hours and couldn't move. I was told that if I did move I would get a bad headache and possibly other side effects. I remember it was a very painful experience.

They told me that I had non-paralytic polio. Yet, I had to learn to walk, sit, stand, and even to go to the bathroom over again. Each time I learned to do something independently, I felt a real sense of joy.

Most of the time I had to just lie in bed, flat on my back. I had no pillow, and my feet were flat up against a footboard. They wrapped my legs in hot packs twice a day, and then I would do exercises. After about one month, they finally told me that I could stand for three minutes. I was so sick of being in bed that I thought three minutes wouldn't be long enough. Well, after standing for one minute, I was ready to lie down again!

I was at Sister Kenny Institute from August until October. I even had my school lessons there. There were seven other girls in the room with me. We were all polio patients and all between 14 and 16 years old. Although we were different ages and religions, it didn't matter. We got to be like a family. We competed with each other for improvements, and we were all very happy for someone who got well enough to go home. I corresponded with some of those girls for several years after leaving the hospital.

I was very thankful that my brother and his wife were able to come and visit me almost every day. My parents were able to come only a few times to visit. I remember one time my dad got a ride on a cattle truck that was going from Evansville to Minneapolis so that he could visit me. A friend brought mom down a few times, but it was such a long trip for them to make. My mother did write to me almost every day though, and I got a lot of mail from my classmates back home. The mail helped with my mental attitude, but this was still a very traumatic time in my life. I didn't really understand the illness; I was 15 years old, and I just wanted to get well and get on with my life.

By October, I had gotten strong enough to walk with Kenny sticks. I could go backwards, and I even walked up stairs. My muscle tests showed some low numbers, but I had a lot of scores in the 5 to 8 range (out of 10). That meant I was well enough to go home. I had to rest and continue to do my exercises at home, but I thought that I was home to stay. However, when I came back in November for a check-up, I hadn't improved. In fact, I had actually lost some of the gains I had made while I was in the hospital, so they didn't let me go home that day. Instead, I had to stay at the hospital!

I was very upset. I had been home, and I had seen some of my friends and my classmates and my family. Now, I was back at Sister Kenny again. The whole thing was difficult for me to accept.

For the next two months, I worked very hard to build up my muscles. I kept telling myself, "There are better days ahead." And finally, with the help of hot packs, hard work, determination, and faith in God, the better days came. I passed my muscle strength tests, and my brother and sister-in-law took me home to Evansville for Christmas. I'll never forget that Christmas. It was the best one of my life!

I went back to Sister Kenny Institute in February for another check-up. This time I had done well, so I was able to return to school. I only went for half the day at first. I was still walking with the Kenny sticks, so someone had to carry my books for me. I was 16 years old now, and I finally felt like I was getting back to a normal life.

By now, people were coming to visit me regularly. Many from my community were eager to help me get back into school and church activities. One of our neighbors had recently lost his wife to cancer. He would come over, and mom would cook him a good meal. He and I played cards and helped each other through these hard times.

By that next summer, I was walking without the sticks. I still needed corrective shoes, and I wasn't able to do many of the normal things that most teenagers do. For instance, I wasn't able to take driver's training classes because my legs weren't strong enough to work the clutch and brakes and gas pedal. There weren't very many automatic transmissions in those days, so I didn't learn to drive until later in life.

It was hard for me to get back into school, church, and community activities again. I wasn't ashamed of using a wheelchair or Kenny sticks when I was in the hospital, but as a teenager I didn't want to be thought of as "different." I couldn't take P.E. because I might have fallen in the shower room. I had a friend who had a weak heart, and we spent a lot of time together as we both had to face similar struggles.

I remember going caroling that next Christmas. I got so cold, and my legs cramped up so badly. I'll never forget how painful that was.

As I think back on that point in my life, I am thankful for Sister Kenny Institute and all their knowledge and care. I was lucky to have gotten the quality treatment that I did. I can't help but wonder though, if I would have suffered less damage had I gotten to Sister Kenny right away.

I am also thankful that I had parents who were willing to work with me and make me do my exercises. I am grateful that I didn't have a more severe case than I did. There always seemed to be someone else who had it worse, and that helped me put my own problems in perspective. Finally, I'm very appreciative of the March of Dimes. My parents didn't have much money, and I'm sure that my medical expenses were very high. But the March of Dimes took care of all my medical bills.

When I reflect on my stages of recovery, I remember being faithful to my hot baths and my exercises. I really pushed myself to gain my strength back, and I delighted in each function I was able to regain. I remember when I was able to raise my leg off of the bed without assistance; I wanted to run out on the street and cheer and tell everyone about my great accomplishment! However, only a person who had polio could have understood my excitement.

It took nine months, but I really rejoiced when I was able to walk again. However, I still fell often, so I couldn't be left alone very much because once I fell, I had difficulty getting up again. I had to slide myself over to a chair or a wall and sort of work my way up.

For the next several years, I went back to Sister Kenny Institute for an annual check-up. They said that I was doing well, and eventually I was medically discharged. I graduated from high school and worked for a year. I then got married and lived what I thought was a relatively normal life.

As I think back on my life now though, I realize that I've always been an over-achiever. I always had to do so much each day just to feel good about myself, and I was so thankful that I could do things again that I could never say "no." Continually overdoing resulted in a lot of physical pain, and I always have needed a lot of sleep. Yet, I have been very active in our family dairy farm, our church, women's group, school, and 4-H. I raised two children and helped care for my aging parents.

Having to work so hard to maintain a normal life eventually caught up with me. In about 1976, I had mononucleosis. It took me so long to recover. If I tried to go back to doing the housework or helping around the farm, I'd be back down again. Finally, after about four months, I was back to normal.

I had an operation on my foot, and the doctor told me it would take about two weeks to recover. Well, six weeks later I was still having problems. When I would get a cold or the flu, it always took me so much longer than other people to get well. It took me a long time to figure out that my problems recuperating from illnesses were due to my having had polio.

When I was about 35 or 40 years old, I started having terrible pain in my joints and muscles. I got tired very easily. I went to the doctor and had x-rays and blood tests. I got some pills and had physical therapy. Nothing helped. One doctor even suggested that my problems were all in my head. He said, "Are you sure you don't just think you have all these problems? You don't look sick, and the tests don't show any problems."

Then in 1988, my husband and I went to a football game in the Twin Cities with my brother and sister-in-law. On the way home we drove by Sister Kenny Institute. My sister-in-law suggested that I should call Sister Kenny and ask them for my old records. She thought that maybe my doctors could get some information from those records that would help them understand my current problems better.

A few days later I called Sister Kenny Institute and asked them if they could send my records from when I had polio in 1956. As I waited for them to find my records, I explained to the person who was helping me that I was experiencing all this new pain, and I was hoping that the records could help explain why. Well, she asked if I had heard about post-polio syndrome. I said, "No, what's that?" She explained that about 30 or 40 years after you had polio, it's like you get it over again. She also helped me get an appointment at the Sister Kenny Post-polio Clinic.

Thinking about dealing with polio over again was more than I could handle. I just fell apart. I called my sister-in-law and told her what I had found out. I also told my family. I cried a lot. I showed my local doctors my medical records and explained about my appointment at Sister Kenny Institute. They again told me that polio was a thing of the past. I said, "Yes, but I'm here now, and I'm living it again!"

I went to Sister Kenny Institute for my appointment and was diagnosed as having post-polio syndrome. I needed to first accept that I had it and then learn to deal with it. At times it is very difficult to think of the future and what it will bring. I don't want to use braces and walkers and wheelchairs again, but I think the hardest thing for me is to have hand weakness. I didn't experience that the first time I had polio, and until your hands start to become weak, you really don't realize how much you use them.

Shortly after being diagnosed with post-polio, I became involved in a research study conducted at Sister Kenny Institute. The study looked at whether people with post-polio could benefit from riding an exercise bike. I was in the "control" group, which meant that I was "inactive" and didn't actually ride the bike. The reason for having the "control" group was so they could compare us to those who actually rode the bike. The study lasted 16 weeks and showed that those with post-polio could improve their cardio-vascular fitness by riding a stationary bike just like people who hadn't had polio. Riding three times a week for about 20 minutes combined with intermittent periods of rest seemed to work the best.

Those of us who were involved in the research were invited to a meeting where we were told about the results. We got to meet the other participants. As I talked to the others, I couldn't believe how much riding the bike had helped. Meeting and talking to others with the same problems also really helped my mental attitude. One of the doctors there (Dr. Owen) was a polio survivor, and it helped to know that he really understood our problems. I felt a sense of mutual support and understanding there which gave me the idea of starting a local support group for polio survivors.

After the study ended, I started to ride a stationary bike. Within about 10 or 12 weeks, I had little or no pain. I started to sleep well again, and I had fewer spells of fatigue. So riding the bike really did help.

I wrote an article about myself and post-polio syndrome for our local newspaper. In that article, I asked if anyone in the area might be interested in starting a support group. The response was very good, and we began a support group that year. We have so many members now that we have split into two separate branches.

We found a lot of people out there who are dealing with unexplained pain and weakness and directed them to Sister Kenny Institute or other medical facilities that know about post-polio problems. I now send out about 50 newsletters for each meeting.

The goal of our group is to reach out to polio survivors and their families and to educate doctors and the general public about post-polio. The first week in June is National Post-polio Week, and this last June (1993), with the help of Sister Kenny Institute, we held a workshop in Fergus Falls. We had a very good turnout. I was interviewed on a local radio station, and we had a breakfast for our local medical group. They responded quite favorably, and now people tell me that doctors from our area have a much better understanding of polio and its late effects.

Also in 1993, I was involved in another research study conducted by Sister Kenny Institute. This study looked at the effect of the drug Mestinon on post-polio symptoms. The medication helps with the secretion of a substance produced by our lower brain that helps to tell our muscles what to do. The polio virus affected the lower brains of many of us who had it.

I have been taking Mestinon for about one year, and I believe it helps me. I feel stronger and have less fatigue. Many of the others who take this medication report similar results.

Even though the Mestinon and riding the stationary bike help, I still have had to change my lifestyle because of my post-polio problems. I have learned to pace myself. I try to avoid getting cold, and I do my exercises. I am no longer able to work in our dairy business, but I keep busy with housework, bookkeeping, crafts, my grandchildren, and church. I have found that helping others with post-polio helps to keep my mind off of my own problems. My faith in God and my family support also help immensely.

I now have braces for both of my legs and both of my hands. I use various adaptive devices to help conserve my energy. My exercises and medication have brought my pain under control. All of this has helped me learn to live with polio the second time around.

Chapter 12

Conclusions

When I began this project three years ago, I did so with only the modest goal of documenting the life experiences of a sample of polio survivors. I had no agenda, no hypothesis that I was trying to demonstrate or examine. I knew little about polio other than the fact that I had it and would have preferred that I had not. I had very little idea of what I might learn about polio and those whose lives were affected by it. I did anticipate, however, that those we would interview were likely to be a diverse group with a variety of experiences and types and degrees of disability. Based on my own experiences, I also expected that most polio survivors would be living ordinary, productive, and reasonably happy lives.

These expectations generally proved to be accurate. Of the individuals whose interviews appear in this book, all but one are or were employed either outside of the home or as homemakers. Nearly all are married, have children, and lead reasonably ordinary home and family lives.

The degree of their disabilities is quite variable. Several, like Marlene Krumrie and Stuart Goldschen, appear to have recovered completely from their acute illness. They have no paralysis, few, if any, post-polio symptoms, and little or no disability. Others, such as Marilynne Rogers and David Kangas, have severe paralysis and have been significantly disabled from the time they first contracted the disease. Still others, such as James Berry and Jennifer Williams, recovered relatively well from their initial illness only to become significantly disabled later in life due to polio's late effects.

Most of those who remember their acute illness recall the classic symptoms of fever, headache, upset stomach, and in some cases, a stiff neck and muscle aches. Several remember having limb weakness or paralysis before going to the hospital. Nearly all believe that they were the only person in their school, neighborhood, or even their entire community to have developed paralytic polio at the time they were ill.

As far as the medical treatment they received, a few remember getting penicillin injections or receiving other sorts of medications. However, nearly all those we interviewed who had polio after 1940 recall being treated with Sister Kenny's method of hot packing, stretching, and manipulation of affected limbs. One might suspect that so many of those we interviewed received the Kenny method because they had been hospitalized and treated in Minnesota. Though this may be true to some extent, even those from other states recalled receiving the Kenny treatment.

Only Richard Owen, who contracted polio in 1940, was treated with the typical pre-Kenny approach consisting of prolonged splinting and immobilization. He is also the only one of our interviewees who recalled being injected with the so called "convalescent serum," an ineffective concoction made from the blood of those who had recently recovered from polio.

Though I had polio in 1953, my treatment was somewhat unusual in that I was not treated with the Kenny method. Rather, I was given injections of curare to reduce my muscle spasms and allow my limbs to be stretched and manipulated. While I have not interviewed other polio survivors who received this treatment, apparently the use of curare was considered a "safe, convenient, and effective" alternative to the Kenny method (Boines, 1952).

By today's standards, many of those we interviewed had hospital stays of incredibly long duration. Several recalled being hospitalized for nearly a year, and Marilynne Rogers told us that she spent more than two years in the hospital. With these lengthy hospitalizations, it is no wonder that many interviewees remember the polio wards as being extremely crowded during the years of major epidemics.

After their release from the hospital, most of those we interviewed attempted to pick up their lives at the point where they had been interrupted by polio. Many, including those who had tutors or received homebound instruction, returned to school and were able to keep up or at least catch up with their classmates. Though architectural barriers presented problems for some of those we interviewed, only Diane Keyser attended a special "orthopedic" school.

Regarding their follow-up treatment, many recall doing exercises and stretching after their release from the hospital. Some remember receiving other forms of treatment such as electrical stimulation and chiropractic care. Perhaps the most unusual form of follow-up treatment was that given to Mary Ann Hoffman. She was given anesthesia and then a physician pounded on her leg until it was black and blue. She remembers the procedure as being called "nerve stimulation." It can only be assumed that the idea behind this "treatment" was to somehow reactivate the motor neurons. Mary Ann doesn't believe the technique to have been successful, and one can only wonder if there was any research to support the use of such a procedure.

Many of those we interviewed had surgery at some point after their initial hospitalization. In fact, those 15 interviewees who reported having surgeries underwent a total of 40 surgical procedures. Additional problems occurred as a result of several of these surgeries, and at least in retrospect, a few appear to have been badly botched. Underscoring the differences between today and the era in which these individuals had their surgical procedures, not one of those we interviewed brought a malpractice suit against a hospital or physician.

In addition to the treatment similarities, there are several other common threads or themes that appear in the interviews. One of these relates to the interviewees' descriptions of their own disabilities and their determination to succeed in spite of them. In reading through the interviews, one cannot help but note the tendency on the part of some to down-play or minimize the extent, or at least the impact, of their disabilities. Jack Dominik's description of his disability is, perhaps, the most extreme example of this tendency. After telling us about paralysis or weakness in all four of his limbs, he added, "Other than that, I don't have any limitations. There were others who had it a lot worse than I did."

Though not addressing the issue as directly, several other interviewees expressed similar perspectives. Many told us that they have never considered themselves to be disabled. Some stated that they cross-country skied, canoed, danced, jogged, or participated in various athletic, recreational, or work-related activities that one might predict would be quite difficult or even impossible for a person with a physical disability. Several believe that their disabilities actually made them become more competitive and determined to succeed.

One might make the case that these attitudes and behaviors are the result of denial, and this may be true for some. However, most of those we interviewed have had 40 or more years to adjust to and learn to cope with their disabilities, and many have few, if any, memories of their lives before polio. They have found ways to do many, if not most, of the things that they needed and wanted to do and have lived good, productive lives in spite of their limitations. Therefore, they tend to view their physical differences as inconveniences that sometimes complicate or make their lives more difficult, but rarely prevent them from accomplishing their goals. Based on the interviews, this perspective seems to be a realistic one.

Growing up in the 1940's, 50's, and 60's probably also played a role in molding the attitudes of polio survivors toward their disabilities. As illustrated in several of the interviews, few accommodations were made during those decades for individuals with physical limitations. Therefore, polio survivors had no choice but to cope as best they could, for if they didn't, they were simply excluded.

Attitudes of physicians and therapists also more than likely contributed to the attitudes of polio survivors toward their disabilities. As Sharon Kimball recalled when she described her first therapist, "She didn't want a whimper or a tear from any of us. We were to be tough and gritty." Long before the Nike commercial, Bob Gurney remembers his therapist telling him, "Don't think about it. Just do it." He did; we all did. Our physicians and therapists expected us to work through the pain and overcome, or at least work around, our disabilities. For the most part, we did.

To some extent, it is possible that these tendencies to minimize the extent of one's disability can be traced back to Sister Kenny and her attitudes and beliefs. As noted in Chapter One, Elizabeth Kenny believed that polio patients needed to "be willed to move paralyzed limbs." Ray Gullickson recalls that she had little sympathy for or patience with those who weren't willing to work to get better, and June Radosovich remembers the prevailing attitude at Sister Kenny Institute to be one emphasizing self-help. "They tried to make you help yourself. They really impressed that on you, that you've got to help yourself." Since Kenny's approach to treating polio patients became so widely accepted, it should not be surprising that her attitudes would also become accepted, not only by the medical community, but by polio survivors themselves.

It is also quite likely that parental behaviors played a prominent role in the development of these attitudes of determination and coping. As noted by Kessler (1966), there are many references in the early literature on physical disabilities regarding the relationship between parental attitudes and those of the child toward his or her disability. Many of those we interviewed described their parents as bound and determined that they would overcome, or at least make the best of, their disabilities. As Pat Zahler noted, "(My father) was determined that there was not going to be anything I couldn't do ... In fact, he said I'd probably do it better!" Pat and many of the others that we interviewed seem to have adopted these same attitudes.

In addition to the importance of parental attitudes, one cannot help but note the frequency with which those we interviewed described incredible amounts of time and energy that parents, particularly mothers, invested in their recoveries. As Sharon Kimball noted, "(Mother) was a trooper through it all. Whatever the doctors said to do, she did." Sharon's mom was certainly not alone. Many of the interviews include accounts of parents staying at the hospital with their children during long hospitalizations, taking on the burdens of home therapy programs, and even constructing adaptive living devices to improve their child's comfort or functioning level. One cannot help but wonder if these same sorts of efforts would still be possible today given the fact that so many children come from single-parent families or families where both parents are employed outside the home.

Though parental support and encouragement were important factors in the processes of recovery and readjustment, no amount of parental effort could shield their children from all potential problems, and many of those we interviewed told us that they experienced some difficulties with social acceptance. This particularly seemed to be the case during the adolescent years. In fact, several interviewees found adolescence to be a very difficult period. Considering the developmental tasks faced by a typical adolescent, this finding is not surprising.

Adolescence is a crucial stage in identity development, and in order to accomplish this developmental task, the adolescent must forge an identity that, at least to some extent, is separate from parents and family. A first step in this process is acceptance by age peers. Craig (1992) and others have noted that physical appearance plays a vital role in this peer acceptance. Craig also noted that adolescents are often rather intolerant of deviations to what they believe to be the norm, be it in behavior or appearance. Therefore, body type and overall appearance become of paramount importance during this period, and many adolescents become quite sensitive about and dissatisfied with some aspect of their appearance. Adolescents with obvious physical deviations certainly must experience these feelings of sensitivity and dissatisfaction more intensely.

A phenomenon referred to by Piaget and others as "adolescent egocentrism" also plays an important role in the behavior of adolescents. As Craig noted, "Adolescents tend to assume that others are as fascinated about them and their behavior as adolescents are about themselves. They may fail to distinguish between their own concerns and the concerns of others" (p. 405). Therefore, adolescents tend to feel that they are continually being watched and often experience anxiety about having their inadequacies discovered by others.

Since these phenomena occur even for those with "normal" bodies, it is certainly not surprising that they may be exacerbated by a physical abnormality. As Sharon Kimball noted during her interview, "Just being 14 is difficult enough, but being in a body cast really complicates things."

Some of those we interviewed told us that they still occasionally feel self-conscious about their physical appearance. However, this is likely to be more a case of minor embarrassment than a major source of anxiety or concern. Actually, it was our perception that the majority of those we interviewed had an overall sense of satisfaction with their current lives, and any left over "scars" seemed to be more physical than emotional. Even those who spoke of childhoods lost due to illness, hospitalizations, surgeries, braces, and disabilities, typically did so with surprisingly little bitterness. The fact that so many of those we interviewed are functioning well speaks volumes for the resiliency of the human spirit and should give optimism to parents who are currently raising a child with a disability or chronic illness.

Unfortunately, many of our interviewees did report having what would appear to be post-polio-related difficulties. Though the exact number of those experiencing these problems is hard to pin down, about one-third have either had a formal diagnosis of post-polio syndrome or appear to have obvious post-polio symptoms. The symptoms most typically reported by this group are quite consistent with those described in the professional literature. They typically began 30 or more years after the acute illness, and include new or increased pain, progressive weakness, and excessive fatigue. Also consistent with the literature, several interviewees experienced difficulty in getting a diagnosis and plan of treatment for their post-polio problems. As Jennifer Williams noted, "I guess what really happened was I diagnosed myself."

Of those reporting significant post-polio problems, some take medications or attempt to manage their symptoms with exercise programs. A few have had to begin using or return to the use of canes, braces, or wheelchairs. Accepting the need for such aids has been, and still is, difficult for some of them. Several told us that in spite of their difficulties with mobility, they have trouble accepting the use of handicapped parking. In fact, just accepting the fact that they are now "disabled" and do have limitations has been very difficult and has required a totally new mind-set, one recognizing that post-polio syndrome is something to be lived with, not overcome. The "just do it" attitude that served Bob Gurney and others in this group so well no longer works. Rather, overdoing and pushing themselves past their limits is now only likely to cause further weakness and make their situations worse. As Jenny Williams noted ruefully:

> ... our parents told us we were just like everyone else, and if we wanted to do something, we could do it. It might be harder for us, but we could do it. I think we just got that in our brains, and it's hard for us to accept that we have limitations now, that there are things we can't do. Our parents always told us, 'You can do it; you can work around it; you're going to get better.' But what I have now is not going to get worked around; it's not going to get any better. In fact, it's probably going to get worse, and that's scary.

In sharp contrast to this group, about another third of those we interviewed does not seem to be experiencing any post-polio problems. They continue to function quite well and report no new pain or weakness. In fact, they appear to be in remarkably good health considering their overall situations.

The remaining third falls somewhere between these first two groups. Though their problems are relatively mild, those in this middle one-third are currently experiencing new pain or other symptoms that may be polio-related. In a few cases, their problems have been diagnosed as being due to arthritis or other known conditions. Some have not sought medical help for their current difficulties, and thus have no diagnosis.

Many of those in this middle group who told us about new pain and other symptoms are in their 50's or 60's, a period of the lifespan when any number of medical conditions may begin to occur. Therefore, based only on their interviews, it is impossible to say with certainty whether any of the individuals in this group have post-polio syndrome. The situation of these interviewees seems to illustrate the difficulties in diagnosing post-polio syndrome, and perhaps sheds some light on the wide variation in the professional literature regarding the prevalence of this condition.

Several of those we interviewed, including some with significant post-polio problems, were able to identify positive outcomes that occurred as a result of their polio experiences. These "silver linings" often related to a perception of increased acceptance of or sensitivity to the problems and needs of others. A few even felt that because of having a disabled parent, their children are more accepting of others who are different from themselves.

Those working in the helping professions often felt that their own disability made it easier for them to gain acceptance from and relate to their handicapped patients or clients. As Gail Bias, a social worker, noted, "I find that handicapped people, especially children, seem to relate to me very well. There's just sort of a natural connection there..."

A few of those we interviewed believed that their having had polio resulted in them becoming better and more serious students. As Dale Jacobson, a dentist, told us, "...having had polio made me realize that I needed to pursue a career in which my physical limitations would not handicap me. I knew rather early on that my real calling would be somewhere in academics, and that was where I needed to put my efforts."

Mary Ann Hoffman and Dick Owen expressed similar thoughts in their interviews. Mary Ann told us that having polio probably resulted in her leaving the rural area where she had grown up and attending college. Dick Owen believes that contracting polio and his subsequent disability were major factors in his becoming a physician. In fact, he stated, "...it's just a fascinating thing to think that perhaps polio changed my entire life's course."

In his book, *A Whole New Life*, Reynolds Price (1994) makes a similar point. Price believes that becoming disabled, be it from an accident or illness, results in us becoming different people who have very different life experiences than would have been the case without our disabilities. Thus, the random event of coming into contact with the wrong person or being in the wrong place at the wrong time changes one's life from that point on and sends it in a totally new direction.

I agree with Price, and like Dick Owen, I've been fascinated by this thought. I have many times wondered what my life would have been like had I not contracted polio in 1953. How did that event change my life? Was it changed for the better or the worse?

The easy answer, of course, would be to say that it was changed for the worse, and I have fantasized over the years about traveling back in time and warning my mother of my impending illness so that she might somehow have prevented it. Yet, given that chance, would I take it? Would any of us whose stories appear in this book want to take our chances on totally living our lives over? Perhaps some would. However, I think that the following passage from Mary Ann Hoffman's interview expresses the thoughts of many of us:

> I've thought this through because I do a lot of work with the grieving process, and if you'd say, 'Well Mary Ann, you'll be able to run and dance and do all sorts of things that you've never been able to do,' I'd say, 'Yeah. that'd be great.' But if I had to go back and not have the same life's journey, I think I'd say, 'No thank you.' It's been 45 years, and I like where I've gone and where I am. I don't like the disability, but I do like my life and the life's journey I've had.

....

So there you have it: the stories of 35 polio survivors and my modest attempts at their interpretation and analysis. I realize others might interpret them differently, and I have no quarrel with that. The stories are, after all, just that--stories. As such, readers can make of them what they will. I also realize that this book only scratches the surface. With about 400,000 polio survivors still among us, that leaves well over 399,000 stories untold. I have no doubt that many of those are remarkable.

References

Albertson, D.L. (1978). *Sister Kenny's legacy.* Minneapolis: Hennepin County Historical Society.

Boines, G.J. (1952). The use of curare in a repository medium in the management of acute poliomyelitis. *American Practice,* Nov., 879-880.

Bradshaw, N. (1989). Polio in Kentucky-from birthday balls to the breakthrough. *Register of the Kentucky Historical Society,* 87 (1), 20-39.

Codd, M.B., Mulder, D.W., Kurland, L.T., Beard, C.M., O'Fallon, W.M. (1985). Poliomyelitis in Rochester, Minnesota. 1935-55: Epidemiology and long-term sequelae: A preliminary report. In Halstead, L.S. & Wiechers, D.D. (Eds.), *Late effects of poliomyelitis* (pp. 121-134). Miami: Symposia Foundation.

Committee (1969). Evaluation of the Kenny treatment of infantile paralysis. *Archives of Physical Medicine and Rehabilitation,* Sept., 531-535.

Craig, G.C. (1992). *Human development.* Engelwood Cliffs, New Jersey: Prentice Hall.

Elmer-Dewitt, P. (1994, March 28). Reliving polio. *Time.* pp. 54-55.

Frick, N.M., & Bruno, R.L. (1986). Post-polio sequelae: Physiological and psychological overview. *Rehabilitation Literature,* 47 (5-6), 106-111.

Headly,J.L. (1995). The latest from the later life effects (LLE) study. *Polio Network News*, 11 (1), 7-8.

Jones, K. (1993). A case for the Salk vaccine. *Saint John's University Symposium: A Faculty Journal*, 11, 23-35.

Jones, D.R., Speier, J., Canine, K., Owen, R. & Stull, A. (1989). Cardiorespiratory responses to aerobic training by patients with postpoliomyelitis sequelae. *Journal of the American Medical Association*, 261 (22), 3255-3258.

Keegan, R.A. (1994). Status of polio in the world today. *Polio Network News*, 10 (3), 3-4.

Kessler, J.A. (1966) *Psychopathology of childhood*. Engelwood Cliffs, New Jersey: Prentice Hall.

La Force, F.M. (1983). The problem of poliomyelitis. In National Council for International Health (NCIH) (Ed.), *New developments in tropical medicine* (pp. 29-33). Washington D.C.: NCIH

Longmore, P.K. (1978, September). Uncovering the hidden history of people with disabilities. *Reviews in American History*, 355-364.

Meier, P. (1972). The biggest public health experiment ever. In J.M. Tanur (Ed.). *Statistics: A guide to the unknown*. (pp.2-13). San Francisco: Holden-Day.

Nathanson, N. (1982). Eradication of poliomyelitis in the United States. *Reviews of Infectious Diseases*, 4 (5), 940-945.

Nathanson, N. & Martin, J.R. (1979). The epidemiology of poliomyelitis: Enigmas surrounding its appearance, epidemiology, and disapearance. *American Journal of Epidemiology*, 110 (6), 672-691.

Owen, R.R. (1990). New problems of polio victims. In Adolph, T. (Ed.), *Health and medical horizons*, (pp. 211-212). New York: Macmillan Press.

Owen, R.R. & Jones, D. (1985). Polio residuals clinic: Conditioning exercise program. *Orthopedics*, 8 (7), 882-883.

Owen, R.R. & Speier, J.L. (1986). *Post-polio news*. (Vol. 1, No. 1). Minneapolis: Sister Kenny Institute.

Owen, R.R. & Speier, J.L. (1986). *Post-polio news*. (Vol. 1, No. 2). Minneapolis; Sister Kenny Institute.

Paul, J.R. (1971). *A history of poliomyelitis*. New Haven: Yale University Press.

Price, R. (1994). *A whole new life*. New York: Atheneum Macmillan Press.

Report: More kids saved from disease (1993, December 21). *St. Cloud Times*. p. 1.

Santoli, A. (1981). *Everything we had*. Ballantine: New York.

Sharief, M.K., Phil, M., Hentges, R. & Ciardi, M. (1991). Intrathecal immune response in patients with post-polio syndrome. *New England Journal of Medicine*, 325 (11), 749-755.

Smith, J.S. (1990). *Patenting the sun*. New York: William Morrow & Company.

Speier, J.L., Owen, R.R., Knapp, M. & Canine, J.K. (1987). Occurrence of post-polio sequelae in an epidemic population. In Halsted, L.S. & Weichers, D.D. (Eds.), *Research and the clinical aspects of poliomyelitis*. (pp. 39-48). White Plains N.Y.: March of Dimes Birth Defects Foundation.

Speier, J., Owen, R., Jones, D. & Seizert, B. (1990). *Sister Kenny Institute post-polio update*. Minneapolis: Sister Kenny Institute.

Taber, C.L. (1970). *Taber's cyclopedic medical dictionary*. (11th Edition). Philadelphia: Davis Company.

Vaccine for polio. (1953, February 9). *Time*, p. 43.

Willis, E. (1979). Sister Elizabeth Kenny and the evolution of the occupational division of labor in health care. *Australian and New Zealand Journal of Sociology*, 15 (3), 30-38.

Yarnell, S.K., Wice, M.B., & Maynard, F.M. (1994). Post-polio syndrome 101: Acute polio and post-polio theories. *Polio Network News*, 10 (4), 1-9.

Young, G.R. (1988). Occupational therapy and the post-polio syndrome. *American Journal of Occupational Therapy*, 43 (2), 97-103.